Carpal Tunnel Syndrome

Relieve Carpal Tunnel Syndrome and Wrist Pain

(The Essential Guide to Understand and Cure Carpal Tunnel Syndrome Permanently)

Eddie Sherrill

Published By **Regina Loviusher**

Eddie Sherrill

Carpal Tunnel Syndrome: Relieve Carpal Tunnel Syndrome and Wrist Pain (The Essential Guide to Understand and Cure Carpal Tunnel Syndrome Permanently)

ISBN 978-1-7779502-4-8

Legal & Disclaimer

Table Of Contents

Chapter 1: What Is Carpal Tunnel Syndrome?

Carpal tunnel syndrome is a situation that influences tens of millions of people every yr. It is an trouble which can motive mild to excessive pain alongside aspect many amazing symptoms and signs and symptoms and it may upward thrust up at any age although it is more commonplace over the age of forty five. Generally speaking, carpal tunnel syndrome can purpose many precise signs and symptoms and signs and symptoms and signs and symptoms and signs however the most not unusual embody problems which incorporates ache, numbness and tingling, commonly within the forearm, hand and hands.

Fortunately, regardless of the truth that there are various unique signs and symptoms, it is also quite clean to benefit a evaluation as there are a series of reliable tests to be had in recent times and other similar conditions are without hassle dominated out.

Although diagnosing Carpal tunnel syndrome within reason uncomplicated, some component this is plenty much less so is the precise purpose of carpal tunnel syndrome. In order to recognize your signs a touch better it does assist to comprehend a chunk more approximately what precisely carpal tunnel syndrome is; this is where in this segment comes in. So, below you may discover a smooth motive behind the query 'what is carpal tunnel syndrome?'.

Carpal tunnel syndrome is also called CTS for brief and it takes its call from the carpal tunnel that lies within the wrist. The carpal tunnel is made from 8 small bones regarded instead fittingly as carpal bones; those 8 bones are what shape the carpal tunnel. This tunnel like shape is reasonably small and it lies on the heel of the hand, maximum of the bones of the hand and the transverse carpal ligament. In smooth phrases, the carpal tunnel lies truely because the decrease wrist.

Within the carpal tunnel lie the flexor tendons and the median nerve; the tendons allow the hands to move nicely and the median nerve controls a few muscle agencies and the sensation in your hand and arms. The wrist actually includes 3 major nerves but it is handiest the median nerve we are going to focus on right right here.

The Median nerve itself is chargeable for touch and enjoy in the course of the palms; it moreover works some of the muscular tissues that control the thumb. The median nerve is the best nerve within the hand this is vital in terms of carpal tunnel syndrome as it's miles surely what reasons it.

The direct reason of Carpal tunnel syndrome is the as a substitute inconspicuous median nerve. It nerve in all fairness huge and it runs via the forearm similarly to the wrist and hand. In reality, it hardly ever reasons problems besides for even as carpal tunnel syndrome arises and this in all likelihood explains why a whole lot of us recognise little approximately it.

Basically, carpal tunnel syndrome arises whilst the median nerve being compressed. When the nerve is squeezed or pinched it's far not able to do its procedure well and this is in which signs and signs and signs and symptoms consisting of ache and tingling rise up.

When the nerve is compressed it could reason pain and aching within the short term and intense numbness or lack of characteristic in the arms if left untreated prolonged-time period; this is why it is so crucial to ensure carpal tunnel syndrome is treated as fast as you purchased a analysis.

So, Carpal tunnel syndrome is due to compression of the median nerve but what reasons the compression of the median nerve itself? Well, compression of median nerve is a result of contamination of the surrounding tendons and tissues that is why anti inflammatory treatments can regularly work properly.

Unfortunately, as everyone is one among a kind, it isn't viable to understand what reasons this infection. Therefore, precisely what compresses the median nerve is often a thriller except you have got suffered a wrist harm or have arthritis. The exceptional factor we're able to do is to cognizance on combatting the symptoms of carpal tunnel syndrome, lessen infection of the encircling region or surgically launch the nerve.

Prognosis and Severity

Generally, the severity of carpal tunnel syndrome can variety from character to man or woman and some be stricken through extra debilitating signs and symptoms and signs and signs and symptoms than others. In most instances even though, if CTS is detected early, signs and symptoms and signs and symptoms can often be dealt with and now and again cured inner six months. The greater extreme carpal tunnel syndrome turns into then the harder it is to treat and the much less possibly it's far that signs and symptoms will disappear.

At this point, it's also in reality virtually worth attempting every treatment desire before resorting to surgical remedy. Overall, Carpal tunnel syndrome is not existence-threatening although it does have a slight to crucial effect on satisfactory of lifestyles.

In most instances, Carpal Tunnel Syndrome is a whole existence situation despite the truth that signs and symptoms can remedy for a period of weeks, months or years in advance than reappearing yet again. The super manner to make sure a advantageous analysis is to maintain doing hand, wrist and finger wearing activities every day, no matter whether or not or not or now not you've got were given any symptoms.

What is the distinction among Carpal Tunnel Syndrome and wrist Pain?

The difference amongst carpal tunnel syndrome and wrist pain is tough to spot as frequently, wrist pain may be so excessive that it feels exactly like carpal tunnel syndrome. The first, most obvious distinction amongst carpal tunnel syndrome and wrist ache is that with wrist ache, the carpal tunnel or the median nerve aren't affected in any manner. Usually, with wrist pain, the Median nerve is in incredible running order, even though it is not feasible to inform this without looking on the nerve itself.

Wrist pain may be very excessive and similar to carpal tunnel syndrome, it may radiate from the wrist right thru to the recommendations of the palms. This ache can be silly, aching or stabbing and it could pretty with out issues come and move for the duration of the day or disappear really in advance than reappearing all over again. If you find which you are affected by ache on your wrist, hand or fingers then it's miles likely that it may be each Carpal tunnel syndrome, tremendous wrist ache from a sprain or bruise or a completely one-of-a-kind situation.

One of the situations that CTS is most typically wrong for is repetitive strain harm (RSI) however in evaluation to Carpal tunnel syndrome, repetitive pressure damage (RSI) is each resulting from strain on the tissues or joints within the wrist. This is usually a end result of repetitive strain and generally takes location if you are over and over moving your wrist or hand in a manner that reasons repetitive strain. Usually, in case you communicate to your doctor or clinical practitioner they'll be able to help determine exactly what you are suffering from.

Short-lived wrist ache

If your wrist ache is brief lived then it is probably innocent and could not need ordinary treatment; it is able to sincerely be which you have sprained a ligament or muscle indoors your forearm, wrist or hand. However, if you find out which you are laid low with normal or regular wrist ache then it's miles in all likelihood that you can be tormented by each different harm. This can be some difficulty from tendonitis to arthritis so, in this case, it's miles incredible to are looking for advice out of your medical health practitioner a good way to discover a evaluation.

Numbness

Another distinction among carpal tunnel syndrome and wrist ache is within the symptoms. Although the symptoms many of the ones problems are pretty comparable, one element you'll commonly not get with wrist pain is numbness. This is because of the fact the 3 principal nerves to your hand and wrist control the feeling to your fingers. Therefore, in case you are suffering from numbness, carpal tunnel syndrome is the most probably perpetrator.

Tendonitis

Tendonitis is regularly compelled with carpal tunnel syndrome and it may every so often be now not viable to tell the 2 conditions apart if you have signs that frequently arise in patients with tendonitis. Tendonitis is generally because of repetitive stress so it's also sensible to assume once more and attempt to asses if or how you can have over exerted your arms and wrists.

If you could pinpoint a time in which you understand you have got been seriously straining your hands or wrists earlier than experiencing pain then it's far much more likely which you are stricken by tendonitis. Often, with tendonitis, your tendons will feel quite tight. This also can be a symptom of carpal tunnel syndrome so it's outstanding to have a systematic professional have a observe your wrists to try to decide precisely what you are tormented by.

Arthritis

Arthritis is each other scenario for which carpal tunnel syndrome can be wrong. In the early tiers of arthritis, symptoms and signs often appear in a single or places and that is regularly the palms, due to this that it could be very easy to diagnose carpal tunnel syndrome in preference to arthritis or the other manner spherical.

Both rheumatoid arthritis and osteoarthritis can each motive ache in the hands and fingers that may mimic carpal tunnel syndrome. Tingling sensations and ache inside the wrist also can make evaluation more perplexing.

Guyon Canal syndrome

Within the wrist, in addition to the median nerve there's additionally the ulnar nerve which passes through what's referred to as the Guyon canal. Symptoms of guyon canal syndrome can seem very much like those obvious in carpal tunnel syndrome even though there are some subtle variations. If you're affected by tingling or loss of sensation to your little finger, ring finger and outer 1/2 of of your palm then it's far in all likelihood you're tormented by CTS in place of Guyon canal syndrome.

Symptoms of Carpal Tunnel Syndrome

Usually, signs and symptoms of carpal tunnel syndrome variety from person to individual and now not honestly each person suffers from the equal signs and signs and symptoms and signs and symptoms. Generally even though, CTS suffers all be by using the usage of numerous stages of pain in addition to tingling and numbness; these 3 signs and signs are characteristic of Carpal Tunnel Syndrome.

If you have not suffered from carpal tunnel syndrome earlier than then it's far likely that your symptoms and symptoms and signs and symptoms will development frequently. It is exceptionally uncommon for moderate or excessive symptoms of CTS to appear and with out caution and it is almost usually a sluggish constructing up in phrases of the severity of signs and symptoms and signs and symptoms. To begin with, signs and symptoms of carpal tunnel syndrome commonly make bigger as a stupid, aching pain inside the wrist or palm of the hand.

This can get up in both palms concurrently or fine in a single hand. In the early degrees of CTS, you can also be via tingling, burning or pins and needles sensations for your wrists and hands. These signs and symptoms usually arise alongside ache within the inner arms and higher palm. Over time, the pain and tingling sensations can boom and numbness can arise along facet a sensation of bruising or swelling below the pores and pores and skin.

The most critical detail to mention here is that even as symptoms and signs can turn out to be excessive if left untreated, there's no reason why you can not perceive your signs and signs and then embark on a treatment path so that you can prevent any extra pain coming your way. Below you could find out a severa listing of symptoms associated with carpal tunnel syndrome. Be fantastic to take a phrase of any of the signs and symptoms you do have so that you can then asses the ones at the same time as growing a assessment.

Carpal tunnel Syndrome is commonly fairly smooth to diagnose and if you are affected by any of the symptoms and symptoms above then it is possibly that you may be tormented by CTS. Of path, even as it is feasible to diagnose your self, it's miles continually absolutely helpful to are trying to find a scientific opinion on the manner to rule out some other conditions. If you'd need to take a look at a manner to diagnose carpal tunnel syndrome then you can flick to chapter 2 where you will be able to find out masses of information on self-analysis.

Common Symptoms of Carpal Tunnel Syndrome:

Tingling inside the hands or hand (common within the thumb, index and middle hands)

Numbness inside the hand or fingers

Weakness within the hand (trouble gripping devices)

General pain or ache within the wrist and hand

Early Symptoms of Carpal Tunnel Syndrome:

If you have were given have been given in no manner suffered from CTS earlier than it's far in all likelihood that within the early degrees, the symptoms and symptoms of CTS may be a long way a extraordinary deal much less excessive than in case you've suffered for an prolonged time period. Below you'll find out a list of the most not unusual signs that appear in the early degrees of CTS.

A sluggish numbness or tingling inside the thumb, index and middle fingers (not the little finger)

Fingers end up numb at night time

The capability to alleviate signs and symptoms and signs through way of shaking your hand or wrist

Numbness or ache becomes worse at the same time as using your hand

Occasional aching pain in your forearm, hand or wrist

More immoderate signs and symptoms of carpal tunnel syndrome:

The signs and symptoms beneath are quite severe and typically stand up when you have been affected by carpal tunnel syndrome for an extended time frame (normally 8+ months). Some of the symptoms are quite uncommon and it is probable that you may suffer from some of the ones signs and symptoms and symptoms and symptoms in region of the all.

A mixture of pain, numbness and tingling in the hand and fingers

A burning sensation In the hand or fingers

Chapter 2: Repetitive Stress

It is typically familiar that folks who use their palms and wrists constantly and repeat the equal movements (e.G., musicians, typists, golfers and so on.) are at better risk of growing Carpal tunnel syndrome. This is likewise referred to as RSI or Repetitive Strain Injury and it's miles perception that again and again shifting the wrist, palms and arms in precisely the equal manner places pressure at the Median nerve.

Some health workers consider that repeated stress to the hand and wrist motives pressure on the median nerve in the lower wrist. This can arise way to repetitive motions together with the usage of a laptop keyboard, playing a musical tool or constantly strolling with vibrating device.

Pregnancy

Due to hormonal modifications, Carpal Tunnel Syndrome is not uncommon sooner or later of being pregnant, particularly at some degree inside the later months. The ache may be treated pretty without problems and signs alleviated with the help of a wrist splint. Most of the time, signs and symptoms and signs and symptoms of CTS disappear honestly after pregnancy.

Menopause

In cutting-edge years, it's far been tested that hormonal modifications ultimately of the menopause can reason Carpal tunnel syndrome. There are some of motives for this however it is usually frequently taking place that within the menopause, the wrist structures emerge as enlarged after which press at the nerve within the wrist.

Family History

Research has showed that if you have a circle of relatives data of CTS, you are an extended way much more likely to boom carpal tunnel syndrome your self in a few unspecified time within the future even though it isn't always constantly the case. Genetically speakme, it is not understood if CTS may be handed thru families regardless of the reality that sort of one in 4 humans be bothered by means of CTS even have a close relative with the circumstance.

Injuries

Injuries to the arm, wrist or hand which include breaks or sprains often growth the chance of carpal tunnel syndrome. This sort of harm can place pressure at the median nerve in the wrist; this which therefore consequences in the debilitating signs of carpal tunnel syndrome.

Arthritis

Rheumatoid arthritis has been installation to boom the risk of affected by carpal tunnel syndrome. This is because of the truth arthritis can inflame the tissues and tendons surrounding the median nerve in the hand. This then outcomes in pressure being located at the nerve itself and consequently causes the symptoms of CTS.

The shape of your wrist

Surprisingly, the shape or length of your wrist can be a factor that will increase the chance of laid low with carpal tunnel syndrome. It is concept that when you have a wrist that within reason small and rectangular regular then it is possible which you are much more likely to expand CTS. Also, if you are quick in stature it's far more likely that there may be an awful lot much less area between the bones and tendons to your wrist which in flip way that compression of the median nerve is much more likely.

Diagnosing Carpal Tunnel Syndrome

Carpal Tunnel Syndrome is normally pretty straightforward to diagnose and you may each have a look at yourself at home thru a sequence of tests or visits your clinical medical doctor or scientific practitioner for an examination. It is normally useful to go to your clinical physician, even in case you are first-rate you're tormented by CTS as they may also be capable of rule out exceptional conditions. If you choose to have a study yourself first that allows you to analyze whether or not you is probably tormented by CTS then there's no harm in examining your self at home first.

There are some of particular tactics to diagnose carpal tunnel syndrome and maximum scientific practitioners pick out initially a simple exam in advance than transferring onto in addition exams. If you need to find out if you might be tormented by CTS then the excellent location to begin is with the aid of truely analysing your signs. To try this, test the symptoms and signs and symptoms phase in monetary smash one and phrase down a few factor that you are stricken by. Keep in thoughts that the three number one symptoms of Carpal tunnel syndrome are:

Pain, numbness or tingling within the wrist, hand or palms.

Symptoms emerge as worse at night time or whilst retaining subjects.

Little Finger Unaffected (the median nerve isn't associated with the little finger)

At domestic wrist exam

These exams are both honest and non-invasive. Because of this, many scientific docs and clinical practitioners use them tests to have a take a look at sufferers and they may be the handiest manner of figuring out whether or not or not or no longer or now not you are suffering from CTS. If you feel now not able to behavior those assessments yourself then you can constantly ask a family member or buddy to help you or alternatively, you can go to your medical doctor.

Tinel's Test

Tinel's check have emerge as advanced and named after Jules Tinel in the early 1900's. For a few years, this test has been used extensively so you can inspect how well the median nerve functions and therefore diagnose carpal tunnel syndrome. In current years, it's performance has been challenged and some consider that it is unreliable as tossing a coin. However, using tinel's test similarly to the opposite exams beneath may be a manner of diagnosing carpal tunnel syndrome and this is often a route that most clinical docs observe.

How to behavior Tinel's Test:

Relax your hand and hold it in the the the front of you with your palm handling upwards.

Use palms or a reflex hammer to gently faucet over the median nerve in the lower wrist. You should position your finger on top of the crease within the wrist, sincerely earlier than the wrist joins the hand.

Tap more than one times over the decrease wrist (commonly five-10 instances will suffice)

In addition to this, you may moreover tap speedy tap the lowest of the hand in which the transverse carpal tunnel lies.

To try this, use hands or a reflex hammer to faucet five-10 times with quite slight but agency pressure. You want to function your fingers no longer inside the centre of the palm but barely more inside the direction of the wrist

Results

You may additionally revel in numbness or tingling sensation similar to pins and needles to your hand, thumb, index finger, center finger or 1/2 of the fourth digit (no longer your little finger). This is considered a effective stop end result and it is therefore in all likelihood that you are stricken by Carpal Tunnel Syndrome.

Phalen's Test

Phalen's test is another non-invasive test that you could do yourself, at domestic. The take a look at itself come to be in the beginning advanced via George Phalen who also devised a series of operations for CTS. Along with Tinel's take a look at, this is one of the most famous techniques of figuring out Carpal tunnel syndrome and it can be performed in addition to the opportunity assessments on this section.

Overall, it has a barely higher fulfillment rate than the preceding take a look at and outcomes in accurate results just over 70% of the time.

How to behavior Phalen's Test:

Hold every of your palms in the front of you and location your fingers collectively so that you form a prayer characteristic.

In order to conduct the check, you want to opposite this prayer feature together with your fingers. To do that, location the backs of your hands collectively in order that they're dealing with in the direction of the ground. Flex your wrists and allow your arms maintain close downwards. There need to be very little hollow the various pinnacle of your wrists.

Hold your palms like this for 1-2 mins.

Results

If you are looking for a super result then the consequences of this check need to be much like that of Tinel's test. If you enjoy tingling, numbness or pain within the thumb, index finger, middle finger or half of of the fourth finger then the prevent end end result of the check is considered first-rate. If you be anxious thru no symptoms in any respect then it is not going that you are laid low with CTS.

Reverse Phalen's Test

As the decision suggests, this take a look at is the alternative of the specific Phalen's check as it consists of retaining the palms in prayer in area of opposite prayer characteristic. This precise check is considered to be beneficial for milder symptoms and signs and symptoms as it's miles more touchy and will increase the strain on the wrist loads extra.

How to conduct opposite Phalen's take a look at:

Begin by means of using protective your palms in the the front of you and place your palms collectively, coping with upwards so you look as despite the fact that you are praying.

There must be very little area amongst your wrists or arms. Hold this characteristic for two minutes.

Results

If you experience any ache or tingling or a few different normal sensations then it's miles likely which you have carpal tunnel syndrome. If your wrist is unaffected then you definately absolutely ought to experience no ache or ache in any way.

Durkan's Carpal Compression Test

This test is greater current as compared to the preceding and it changed into superior inside the early nineties as an alternative, barely extra moderen model of Tinel's test. It has been proven to be among 87 and 91% accurate in diagnosing Carpal Tunnel Syndrome.

How to conduct Durkan's Test:

Begin thru maintaining your hand in the front of you collectively along with your palm handling up and your wrist exposed.

Using your thumb, press down onto your lower wrist on the factor wherein your wrist meets your hand and above in which the median nerve lies.

Hold your thumb down with business enterprise strain for 30 to 60 seconds.

If you need, you could moreover circulate your thumb slightly lower down and vicinity strain on the lower hand, in fact to the thing of the ball of your thumb. Hold for the identical quantity of time.

Results

During this test, if you revel in any pain, tingling or numbness within the thumb, index finger, middle finger or half of of the fourth finger then it is probable you're laid low with Carpal Tunnel Syndrome.

Chapter 3: Hand Elevation Test

The hand elevation test is a few other current take a look at that is designed to installation whether or not or no longer or now not the median nerve within the wrist is being compressed. Although it isn't always extensively used, this test is idea to be accurate round eighty% - 89% effective the majority of the time.

How to behavior a Hand Elevation Test:

Hold your affected hand above your head as and acquire as high as you can without straining. Try to stay fairly comfortable and ensure that your palm is going through forwards and your arm instantly.

Hold this feature for 2 to a few mins.

Results

If you enjoy any ache, numbness or tingling then it's far possibly that you may have CTS. Again, if any signs and symptoms and signs and symptoms and symptoms of CTS appear sooner or later of the test then it's far taken into consideration a quality cease end result; this can help to diagnose Carpal tunnel syndrome.

Other Tests

Occasionally, Carpal tunnel syndrome can be mistaken for a few trouble without a doubt one-of-a-kind and outcomes from Phalen or Tinel's tests can on occasion be inconclusive; this is wherein opportunity kinds of attempting out are to be had. If each you or your doctor are suffering to verify a prognosis of CTS because of suspected fake fine exam effects or various, unusual signs and symptoms and signs and symptoms then you may undergo one of a kind exams as a way to verify Carpal Tunnel Syndrome.

These assessments are in no way really crucial however they'll be very useful and dependable if you're struggling to get maintain of a evaluation of Carpal Tunnel Syndrome. The maximum well-known assessments for Carpal Tunnel Syndrome are an EMG (Electromyogram) or a Nerve Conduction Test. These exams offer definitive consequences and they may be a fantastic possibility if, even after present procedure non-invasive checks, you are however uncertain whether or not or no longer or no longer or not you are suffering from CTS.

Nerve Conduction Study

A nerve conduction have a study is a reasonably sincere, non-invasive check and it's far frequently used to diagnose carpal tunnel syndrome. During a nerve conduction have a have a study, small electrodes are placed onto the pores and skin of your hand and wrist. These electrodes are attached to a tool which then proceeds to ship a small surprise via the electrodes and into your pores and pores and pores and skin. This wonder pursuits to attain the median nerve inside your wrist and the give up stop result goals to set up how speedy the electrical impulses reach the nerve itself.

Overall, this check objectives to set up if there can be any damage to the median nerve inside the wrist and it's far very rare for suffers of carpal tunnel syndrome to return lower again with ordinary effects; this is why the check is so effective for diagnosing CTS.

EMG

An EMG is a completely dependable manner and it's far extremely good for every diagnosing CTS and ruling out a few specific extra sinister situations. However, an EMG isn't frequently used to diagnose

CTS as in most times, nerve conduction studies and non-invasive tests are enough to confirm a diagnosis.

During an EMG, very small needles are inserted into the muscle mass of the hassle region. The needles are very small and thin and commonly produce little ache. These needles are then used to diploma how properly the muscle groups reply to stimulation. Often, muscle twitches are produced due to this test and people twitches are used to degree how properly the median nerve is functioning and consequently, how seriously it's far being compressed.

X-RAY

X- rays aren't strictly used for diagnosing carpal tunnel syndrome but they may be useful for disposing of other situations in case your medical doctor's isn't definitely certain what's causing your troubles. For instance, xrays can regularly be beneficial for examining the hand and wrist in masses more element as you can see the bone structure very simply. Usually, through an x-ray a scientific practitioner can select up on any vintage injuries causing issues similarly to arthritis or one of a kind wrist problems.

Ultrasound

An ultrasound is a reasonably unusal way of diagnosing carpal tunnel syndrome and it's miles a way usually used if CTS is inflicting particular troubles. An ultrasound is particularly beneficial for searching at the size and structure of the median nerve in the wrist and as it in all fairness quick, clean and painless it can be very beneficial.

What to do in advance than treating Carpal Tunnel Syndrome

It is going without pronouncing that in advance than you start to deal with carpal tunnel syndrome, it is in truth useful (however no longer important) to have an respectable medical prognosis out of your clinical health practitioner or each exceptional scientific professional. Of route, this isn't truely important however it is critical as you could have an underlying medical situation or a few other trouble in an effort to bypass disregarded and untreated in case you maintain to address it as CTS.

Before delving into each stopping and treating CTS, it permits to have an concept of the severity of your symptoms. Usually, the amount of strain at the median nerve can variety drastically and this may determine how excessive your signs and symptoms and signs and symptoms are. If you're suffering from pretty mild signs and symptoms and signs and symptoms and are consequently capable of preserve your life with out an excessive amount of interruption then your treatment plan may be special to that of a person laid low with extra excessive, life-restricting signs and symptoms.

Here you may discover a symptom severity scale questionnaire. As stated, it's miles designed to evaluate how terrible your symptoms and symptoms and signs are so that you can devise a remedy plan spherical this. The plan underneath has been designed with the techniques of Levine DW, Simmons HP and Koris MJ in mind.

How to evaluate the severity of your signs and symptoms and symptoms and symptoms

Symptom Severity Scale

Key   1= Never   2= Mild   3= Moderate/Medium   four=Often Severe and pretty lifestyles-proscribing   5= Very Often/ severe and lifestyles-limiting

1.   How excessive is your hand or wrist pain eventually of the day?

2.   How intense is your hand or wrist pain at night time time on the equal time as in mattress?

three. How often has hand or wrist ache woken you up at night time time time throughout the beyond four weeks?

4.   How often do you be afflicted by wrist or hand ache each day? (1 = little 5 =constantly)

five.   How frequently you be stricken via numbness on your wrist or hand?

6.   How regularly do you be anxious thru tingling or pins and needles on your wrist or hand?

41

7.   Do you be   through problem gripping or dealing with gadgets?

eight. How regularly do your signs and symptoms interfere with each day lifestyles (writing, handling objects, doing chores, strolling and so on)

The consequences of this take a look at are quite self-explanatory however though, this test is frequently very useful in admitting your symptoms and signs and symptoms to yourself. Often, quite a few us have a propensity to neglect about or try and neglect approximately the severity of our signs and symptoms and it isn't till analysing them on a scale of 1-five which you understand how plenty CTS is affecting you.

Results

If you have got scored in maximum instances four's or five's then your signs and signs are at the very extreme prevent

42

of the spectrum and also you need to ensure that you recall all remedy options similarly to exercising your wrists, fingers and hands. If you have got scored at the whole 2's or 3's then your signs and symptoms and signs are mild and in case you've scored in the critical 1's and multiple's you then definately are quite lucky as your signs and signs and symptoms seem like pretty mild and without problem treated.

How to Prevent Carpal Tunnel Syndrome

Preventing carpal tunnel syndrome can be hard truly due to the reality that each person can growth it at any element in their lives. However, what you can do is lessen the risk of developing CTS by the usage of changing high quality conduct and adapting your way of life. Preventative measures are specifically beneficial in case you are already at risk of developing Carpal tunnel, for example, in case you are pregnant, going thru the menopause or have arthritis.

Here you'll find out a list of the most not unusual and powerful preventative measures. All of the topics under had been showed to either make a distinction to or save you carpal tunnel syndrome from growing. It is crucial to say which you without a doubt don't need to comply with the entirety below all of the time however try to adapt your life-style in which critical.

Chapter 4: Effective Preventative Measures

1.   If you use your fingers masses and interact in repetitive motions the usage of your fingers, arms or wrists regularly then the extraordinary element you can do is to relaxation your arms every now and then. If you spend your days on foot, vibrating heavy equipment, gambling musical gadgets or typing then try to take a three-five minute damage every so often in which you can wrest you wrists and arms sincerely.

This will assist to alleviate the strain you placed on your wrist and therefore avoid compressing the median nerve. In addition to this, it is also actually useful to warmness up your fingers and hands before embarking on a repetitive project for an prolonged time body. You can test the segment under for a few exercise mind.

2. Keep your palms warmness

Although it has not been observed why, there may be a hyperlink among cold palms and CTS. It is belief that this is because of the reality your arms are much more likely to grow to be stiff and painful if your palms turn out to be cold for longer periods of time. Whenever you could, try to preserve your arms warmth with the beneficial useful resource of wearing gloves or deliver a hand hotter with you spherical with you.

three. Don't placed too much stress for your arms

The reason of CTS is pressure on the median nerve so it makes sense to keep away from immoderate strain even as the usage of your fingers. Often, it's far very easy to apply your hands forcefully even if performing ordinary duties and this can not simplest purpose pressure on the median nerve however moreover motive extraordinary situations as properly.

If you find which you press very tough on keyboards or distinct controls or write gripping your pen tightly and urgent hard then it's miles crucial to try to alleviate the strain you are placing to your fingers. Whenever viable, attempt to alleviate your grip and use moderate but business enterprise pressure at the same time as using system and finishing responsibilities.

As lengthy as you try and take be aware of even as your fingers are hurting or aching from the quantity of pressure you use, you are midway there besides.

4.   Support your wrist and hands

If you already be through slight wrist pain or kind 2 Repetitive stress harm then it's miles virtually well worth thinking about using ergonomic system to manual your wrist and fingers. Of direction, it is going without pronouncing that you can constantly use ergonomic system even if you aren't stricken by signs and symptoms although it's also at the identical time as symptoms and signs occur that humans appearance to exchange their behavior and assist their arms and wrists.

Ideas

Adjust the tension of your keyboard so that you can press the keys a great deal less complicated, while not having to use excessive stress.

Purchase a wrist rest for your keyboard and mouse mat. This will lessen the quantity of stress located to your wrists and permit your palms to lighten up as you type and use a mouse.

Invest in an ergonomic keyboard. There are a big range of ergonomic keyboards to be had to pick out out from. Most are slightly first rate in phrases of format but all of them relieve strain at the wrist and hands on the same time as typing.

5.   Correct your posture

It can also moreover sound excellent however having accurate posture is virtually a manner of stopping carpal tunnel syndrome. This is because of the truth accurate positioning of the body can useful aid drift and relieve stress placed on positive areas of the body. Therefore, there is probably an awful lot much less pressure located at the median nerve and the blood might be capable of circulate extra freely through the wrists, arms and palms. Below you will find out a few pointers for proper posture.

When sitting down, preserve your ft on the ground or vicinity them on a foot relaxation.

Your elbows need to be alongside your body and your wrists right now always.

When sitting and status keep your decrease lower back as right away as viable and keep away from slouching.

Preventative hand carrying events

Another manner you can prevent carpal tunnel syndrome is to stretch the muscle groups on your wrist and hand each day or earlier than sporting out a mission that includes repetitive movement or the usage of vibrating system. These varieties of hand sports activities sports are never critical but if you supply them out effectively as little as as quickly as an afternoon then it is able to lessen the strain on the median nerve inside your wrist quite significantly.

Most of the hand and finger physical games below art work by way of using the usage of stretching the muscle groups inside the wrists, palms, palms, neck and shoulders. This improves the blood flow to the ones areas and releases the strain positioned on the muscle corporations, nerves and in the end, the median nerve inside the hand which consequently prevents CTS.

Finger Warm Up carrying events for repetitive obligations

These carrying sports are pretty smooth and don't take too much time the least bit. They are designed to warmness up your wrists, hands and arms to reduce the pressure located on the nerves and muscular tissues. Ideally, at least this shape of sports activities need to be completed in advance than repetitive responsibilities which include writing, typing or playing an tool.

1.   Finger Warm Up

Hold your hand in the front of you along facet your palm going thru away.

Starting together together with your little finger, bend each finger backwards as a ways as is snug. Ensure which you do not motive yourself any ache.

Repeat this with every palms and then bend every finger beforehand as an extended manner as is snug.

2.   Hand and finger Warm Up

Place your hand in order that it's far flat inside the the front of you and resting on a desk or special flat surface.

Keep your palms flat on the table and raise each one, beginning together along with your thumb, as an extended way as you locate is comfortable.

Once you've finished, repeat this with the aid of lifting each finger all over again however this time beginning together along with your little finger. Repeat with each palms.

Rest your arms for five -10 seconds.

Start alongside facet your palms flat at the table yet again and grade by grade unfold all your arms aside actually so there is an equal hole among every finger. Spread them aside as far as you could after which bring your hands lower back to a ordinary function.

Repeat this workout with each fingers twice.

Exercises for repetitive responsibilities

1.   Shake each of your fingers backward and forward, promptly however now not too forcefully for 30 - 60 seconds.

2.   Twist your wrists spherical in a spherical motion for 30 - 60 seconds.

three. Squeeze your shoulder blades together and roll your shoulders up and down for 30 - 60 seconds.

Wrist Prevention Exercise 1

1.   Begin thru growing a loose fist at the aspect of your hand and ensure your hand doesn't end up tight and clenched.

2.   Position your fist simply so it's far going through towards you, palm up.

3.   Use your exclusive hand to press in opposition for your fist with a touch strain but now not plenty that it is painful. Try to stand up to the force pressing down to your fist. Hold this for 8 seconds.

4.   Next, turn you fist in order that your palm going through a long way from you.

five. Take your particular hand, palm going via upwards and area your fist in the direction of your palm. Press down at the aspect of your fist so you can sense a piece strain for your fisted hand. Hold this for 10 seconds.

Wrist Prevention Exercise 2

1.   Hold your arm loosely but without delay within the the the front of you as despite the fact that you are assignment for some thing and keep your elbow together with your special hand. Ensure that your palm is going through downwards.

2.   Bend your wrist downwards so your palms are toward the floor and preserve for two seconds. Then boom your wrist in order that your arms are pointed inside the direction of the sky and keep for two seconds.

3.   Repeat this motion and bend your wrists up and down quite speedy for 30 seconds.

Wrist Prevention Exercise three

1.   Hold your palms in the the front of you and then bend your elbows just so

your arms come together and shape a prayer function. You elbow ought to be positioned far from you and your arms collectively without any hole among your wrists or palms.

2.   Keep your palms together and gently lower your hands toward the floor. Ensure your arms are together and in prayer characteristic usually. You should sense a mild stretch on your wrists and forearms.

three. Once you have got were given stretched your palms as a long way as cushty (this is normally round hip peak), keep the position for five seconds.

four. Bring your arms again up to your chest and repeat the previous step five instances.

Treatment for Carpal Tunnel Syndrome

There are many specific remedies available for carpal tunnel syndrome and counting on the severity of your signs and symptoms; these treatments can variety from physiotherapy proper through to surgical remedy. In current, carpal tunnel syndrome can be effectively treated and signs and symptoms and signs and symptoms and signs and symptoms decreased extensively thru following a non-invasive remedy plan. As with some element, it simply lets in to diagnose or treat carpal tunnel syndrome early as it could notably enhance your outlook.

Usually, if carpal tunnel syndrome is diagnosed early then you could use very moderate, much less time eating types of treatment as symptoms and signs are plenty much less prominent. This consists of moderate, quick sports activities designed to be finished some times an afternoon. However, if signs and signs are greater extreme then you could have to combine carrying sports activities with unique kinds of non-surgical remedy.

The most invasive treatment for carpal tunnel syndrome is each open or endoscopic surgical operation and it's far simplest carried out as a closing inn and in case you are stricken by very extreme pain.

It is sizeable that the exceptional form of treatment for Carpal tunnel syndrome is a aggregate of hand and wrist carrying occasions alongside side different styles of non-surgical treatment. In addition to enhancing the signs and symptoms of CTS via wrist and hand sports activities (you'll find lots of those bodily sports in the next phase) you can moreover lessen your signs and symptoms with special kinds of nonsurgical treatment.

Chapter 5: Wrist Splinting

A wrist splint might be the maximum well-known way of decreasing the pain because of CTS and it is able to be used first, earlier than attempting each other form of treatment. They are generally designed to in shape around your wrist, lower arm and part of your hand a good way to preserve your wrist at a independent perspective.

This reduces the stress at the carpal tunnel and median nerve which in turn reduces signs such as pain and tingling on the same time as you are wearing the splint. As wrist splints reduce the motion of your wrist, they'll be hard to put on at some stage in the day if you need to move your fingers constantly.

In this situation, it's miles not unusual to actually put on a splint at night time time because it maintains the wrist in the correct feature and decreases pain that might often interrupt sleep. Sometimes, in case you are tormented by moderate signs and symptoms and signs and signs and symptoms, wearing a wrist splint can significantly lessen or maybe treatment symptoms and signs and symptoms even as worn for a length of weeks.

NSAID'S (Nonsteroidal anti-inflammatory pills)

Although the time period nonsteroidal anti-inflammatory drugs sounds very complex, it really truly technique over the counter anti-inflammatory drugs together with aspirin and ibuprofen. If you aren't best suffering from pain and tingling however infection as properly then NSAID'S can be an outstanding alternative. Unfortunately, NSAID'S don't reduce stress on the median nerve however they do paintings to lessen infection and therefore ache.

Basically, capsules which includes aspirin and ibuprofen block the substances that dilate the blood cells which purpose ache and irritation. On a short-time period basis, NSAID's can paintings to reduce ache and infection but they'll be now not encouraged for long term use as they could reason issues. Therefore, this shape of ache reliever ought to only be used while vital and not as a long time solution.

Corticosteroids

There are styles of corticosteroids, the number one is corticosteroid injections and the second is corticosteroid tablets which is probably orally administered. Both types of steroids art work nicely no matter the fact that there are diffused variations most of the 2.

Corticosteroid injections artwork by the usage of way of shrinking the swollen tissue within the wrist and hand and consequently relieve any stress positioned within the median nerve within the hand. This sort of steroid injection works thoroughly in most sufferers even though it is a reasonably drastic desire.

Generally, this type of remedy is assumed to provide brief time period pain treatment as in maximum sufferers, signs and signs and symptoms recur interior 13 months. Steroid injections are normally limited to a few in step with yr as in any other case, they will be able to purpose complications and factor results which includes woke up tendons and nerve infection which make signs and signs of CTS worse.

The less well-known approach of Corticosteroid treatment is a course of pills. A low dose of corticosteroids may be prescribed via your doctor. The course normally lasts round 1 -2 weeks that permits you to avoid any complications associated with lengthy-term steroid use. Oral Corticated drugs aren't as broadly used as steroid injections clearly because of the truth relief is brief-lasting and typically best lasts 2 -three months.

Ultrasound

Ultrasound treatment is any other opportunity that gives extra short term than long time advantage although it stays a possible treatment opportunity. In assessment to exceptional types of remedy, ultrasound treatment for Carpal tunnel syndrome in all fairness new even though it has been confirmed to be quite powerful at supplying short-time period alleviation.

To deal with Carpal Tunnel Syndrome, an ultrasound is used to direct immoderate frequency waves at the lower wrist in which the median nerve lies. These waves paintings to reduce infection of the tissue within the wrist and therefore lessen the compression of the median nerve. Usually, round 15 to twenty training of ultrasound treatment are desired at the manner to lessen signs for a short time period.

It is vital to mention that the super shape of treatment for carpal tunnel syndrome isn't always usually one single remedy together with ultrasound of steroids, however as an opportunity a aggregate of treatments. Most humans locate that the single simplest way of decreasing ache and soreness is in reality to mix numerous topics and confirm what works for you.

For example, many discover that combining a brief term route of steroids with each day hand wearing sports activities works very well as it reduces pain in the brief time period while the sporting sports paintings to relieve signs and symptoms and signs and signs within the prolonged-time period.

Exercises for Carpal Tunnel Syndrome and wrist pain

It is normally popular that wrist, hand and finger bodily sports are one of the splendid strategies to reduce the symptoms of carpal tunnel syndrome and wrist ache. Most physical video games art work in slightly unique methods however in state-of-the-art, they paintings to alleviate the pressure on the median nerve via each stretching and exciting the encircling areas.

They furthermore relieve symptoms and symptoms of stylish wrist pain by the use of using stretching the muscle agencies, tendons and tissues. There are many one in all a kind carrying sports to choose from and they are all physiotherapy based totally definitely absolutely because of this that they will be perfectly strong and aren't possibly to make your signs and symptoms worse. In addition to this, all sporting sports for carpal tunnel are designed so they don't require any unique device; which means that that that you can resultseasily adapt each workout into your every day lifestyles with out a whole lot problem.

Overall, if you are laid low with moderate to slight Carpal Tunnel Syndrome then there may be no reason why you can not beautify your signs and symptoms extensively thru manner of exercise your wrists, arms and hands.

Most carrying sports (inclusive of those under) for CTS and wrist ache were designed via physiotherapists and examined by way of method of every researchers and sufferers. Below you'll find out a sequence of wearing activities designed to seriously lessen the signs and symptoms of carpal tunnel syndrome. As with any form of workout, it is awesome to start of slowly and constructing up in preference to overdoing it as this could simplest make your signs worse.

If you be afflicted by RSI or every other similar sort of ache then it is greater important than everyday to begin of progressively as you don't need to motive any similarly harm. Remember to keep topics gentle. To start with you need to start by means of way of doing those wearing activities in advance than you start the use of your hands for responsibilities that stress your wrist or purpose you more ache.

You need to moreover attempt to finish the ones bodily video games round 2 times in keeping with day for 5 minutes or so after which boom to 3-4 instances consistent with day for an extended term.

Exercise 1 – Simple Wrist Bend

This exercise is fairly easy and pleasant if you've in no way tried to exercise your wrists or palms in advance than. Ideally, you must do that workout more than one instances an afternoon and then building up at the same time as you could.

Good for: Strengthening and enhancing flexibility in the wrists

Rest you elbow on a flat ground together along with your higher arm and hand positioned vertically.

Begin through bending your wrist in advance, hold your pinnacle arm definitely immediately and bend your hand forwards as a long way as is comfortable.

Bend your wrist lower back towards you actually so it is at once again.

Next, bend your wrist backwards just so your hand is achieving inside the route of your better arm as your wrist actions. Bend it lower back as far as is snug and go again your wrist to its ordinary function all over again.

Repeat those steps with both arms 5 instances in succession and attempt do three gadgets of 10 repetitions once you have got built up.

Exercise 2 – Wrist Resistance Exercise

This exercising is extremely good for each attractive and stretching the muscle groups in the forearm and wrist. It furthermore in quick reduces the strain in the wrist as awesome muscle businesses are operating to stand as much as the strain. With this exercise, it is important now not to overdo the strain you vicinity to your hand as this may cause damage. Keep in mind that you need to be slight but simply forceful sufficient to prevent your hand from growing.

Good for: Strengthening the wrist and arms and quick relieving nerve pressure.

Place your proper hand on a flat ground after which put your unique give up the pinnacle of it. Ensure that your different (left) hand does no longer cover the suggestions of your palms or knuckles.

Press down gently together together with your left hand and at the same time, try to push your proper hand upwards. Both of your fingers must be searching for to stand up to the strain of the possibility and also you need to feel the muscles for your wrist and forearm jogging.

Hold this stress for five seconds first of all and characteristic a 5 2nd smash earlier than continuing to copy the workout three times with each hand. You can then glide onto 6 to 10 times with every hand at the same time as you enjoy snug with this exercising.

Exercise three – Standing Wrist Bend

This workout is every other model of exercising one but it is completed repute up as a substitute. This approach that the muscle agencies on your forearms and wrists get extra of a chunk out as it calls for a touch greater strength to hold your hands out within the the front of you. As always, perform this exercising lightly and avoid bending your wrists to the point that it is uncomfortable; you want to exceptional enjoy a mild pull or stretch.

Good For: Flexing the wrists and hands

Bend with the resource of way of recognition along with your hands right away out within the the front of you and ensure your arms and fingertips are pointing forwards.

Extend every of your wrists so that you pull each hand upwards. Your palms ought to be within the same role as they might if you have been doing a hand stand. Once you've bent your wrists upwards as an extended way as is cushty, hold the area for five seconds.

Relax and straighten your wrists. Position your fingers without a doubt so they're held far from you all over again.

Hold your fingers out in the front of you as in advance than and bend your wrists downwards, towards the floor. Bend your wrists as a protracted manner as is cushty and keep this characteristic for 5 seconds.

Relax and straighten your wrists again and shake your wrists lightly back and forth.

You can repeat this manoeuvre three – 5 instances initially and then as many as 15 instances while you experience you are ready.

Exercise 4 – Standing hand and wrist flex

This workout is a mixture of hand and wrist stretches. It is nice for while you've come to be snug with the preceding physical video video games and need to move onto a few issue a hint more advanced.

Good For: Strengthening the arms and flexing the wrists

Begin through using maintain your palms right away inside the front of you and permit your fingers to lighten up.

Ensure that your palm is dealing with down, in the direction of the floor and lightly bend your hand down the use of your wrist joint.

Use your other hand to drag your stretched hand in the direction of your frame very lightly. Continue this until you feel a subtle stretch (however no pain!) and keep for 10 – 15 seconds.

Release your hand and straighten your wrist. Allow your hand to lighten up.

Begin all yet again together with your hand inside the the front of you and your palm dealing with in the route of the ground. Begin to bend your wrist in order that your hand factors inside the air.

Then use your contrary hand to pull it in the route of you gently. Stop even as you feel a subtle stretch and hold for 10 – 15 seconds.

Return you hand to its normal characteristic and loosen up.

Continue this with both palms and repeat 3 instances with every hand. You can increase this to 5 – 6 times at the identical time as you feel you're equipped.

Exercise five - Wrist Flexor Stretch

This exercise may be very popular with physiotherapists and it truly works very well for plenty sufferers tormented by Carpal Tunnel Syndrome. This exercise is designed to boom the motion of your wrist and stretch your muscle groups simply so they do not press at the median nerve.

Good For: Flexing the palms and wrists

Begin by means of the use of way of retaining your right arm right away inside the the front of you together alongside your palm facing upwards, in the direction of the sky.

Keep your elbow and arm at once and corporation and preserve onto the fingers of your proper hand at the side of your unique hand.

Allow your wrist to move and gently man oeuvre your right hand downwards, within the route of the floor. Use your unique (left) hand to tug your wrist lightly downwards without causing any ache or pain.

Stop at the equal time as you sense a snug, mild stretch and keep the placement for 10 – 15 seconds.

Repeat the preceding step collectively collectively with your left hand. Hold your hands collectively with your proper hand and gently pull your wrist downwards yet again following exactly the identical suggestions as before.

Repeat this workout three-5 times with every hand and increase to six-8 instances while you experience more cushty.

Exercise 6 – Standing arm rotation

This workout is designed to stretch the muscle tissues to your arm and forearm. This can assist to enhance the energy of the muscle groups surrounding the median nerve which in the end outcomes in less stress round this place. With this workout, make sure which you maintain you better arm surely proper now and unmovable and only pass the limbs underneath your elbow.

Good For: Stretching the hands and fingers

Hold your arm within the front of you along aspect your elbow at your facet. Your arm must be bent in a ninety diploma mind-set. Ensure that your palm is handling downwards, closer to the floor.

Gently, begin to rotate your hand, wrist and forearm upwards in order that ultimately, you palm is dealing with up.

Hold your arm and hand in this role for 10 seconds.

Begin to rotate your arm, wrist and hand once more into its regular function just so your palm faces closer to the ground yet again.

Repeat this workout 5-10 instances.

Exercise 7 – Wrist Pressure Exercise

This exercising is good for building energy to your wrists. It is a great idea to strive this work out a couple of weeks while you've started stretching and exercising your arms as you don't want to cause yourself any discomfort.

Good For: Strengthening the wrists

Begin via standing up and place your palms on a flat ground. Make certain that the floor you're leaning on allows your palms to increase completely as though it is too immoderate you'll now not be able to absolutely this exercising successfully.

With your hands flat, gently bend your wrists in order that your arms are flat at the ground and your hands are vertically located within the the front of you. With your frame, location slight stress to your wrists so you are able to guide some of your frame weight. Hold the region for five seconds.

Then turn both of your wrists and arms just so your fingertips are facing in the path of your frame.

Exercise eight – Standing arm extension exercising

This exercise is a notable for stretching and increasing the limbs. It not first-rate works to stretch the hands however furthermore gently stretches the wrists and flexes the palms as nicely. This workout is a honestly suitable all-rounder.

Good For: Stretching the lower fingers, wrists and arms.

Begin through standing an hands- length some distance from a wall or door.

With your arm actually prolonged, area your fingertips towards the wall and gently bypass your wrist in order that your palm little by little lies flat in opposition to the wall.

Lift your palm from the wall and pull your hand backwards just so your fingertips are in opposition to the wall all all over again.

Continue this 10 -15 times in a smooth motion and increase to twenty times whilst you sense succesful.

Exercise nine – Standing arm and wrist rotation

This is some other extremely good exercising for stretching your palms further to your wrists. It works properly to relieve stress on the median nerve in the long term really as it stretches and flexes particular muscular tissues. Once you've spent a few weeks training the opposite bodily sports, make sure to do this one every day.

Good For: Stretching the forearms and wrists

Stand so you are an arm's duration a ways from a wall or door.

Place your palm closer to the wall simply so your fingers are facing upwards, in the direction of the sky. Your hand need to be positioned at 12 zero'clock. Gradually twist your hand, beginning by means of the usage of way of twisting your wrist and then your forearm and better arm truly so your hands rotates spherical to six o'clock.

Hold your hand right right right here for 5 2nd and rotate your hand, wrist, forearm and higher arm decrease again to the 12 o'clock feature over again.

Repeat this three times after which waft onto your one-of-a-type hand. You can drift onto 5-6 repetitions with each hand at the same time as you sense cushty.

Exercise 10 – Hook Fist Exercise

This workout can be very famous with each physiotherapists and patients of CTS because it simply works to relive signs and symptoms. It is a specially proper idea to work out this workout if you suffer from painful, numb or tingling arms as it really works and stretches the arms and the palm of the hand.

Good For: Maintaining flexibility in the arms and hand

Place your palms on a flat floor simply so your arms face upwards. Ensure that your fingers are open and relaxed.

Gently start to curl the higher part of your knuckles (or 1/2 of your finger) inwards so that you create a partial fist. Ensure that you don't curl all your knuckles right proper right here.

Return your palms to their conventional, open positon.

Next, bend all your hands and maintain them straight away till you shape a straight away fist. Squeeze your arms gently for two -3 seconds and release. Return your hands to their regular position.

You can repeat this exercise 5 – 10 times with each hand – it's miles as masses as you whether or not or now not you exercising both fingers on the same time or one after the other.

Exercise eleven – Standing Fist Exercise

This workout is excellent for all regions of the fingers and wrists and it improves energy in addition to flexibility. You can also complete this exercising barely in a few other way with the useful aid of a foam ball. You'll discover a more superior model of this in some time on this section.

Good For: Strengthening the fingers and wrists.

Hold your proper hand in the the front of you collectively together with your palms directly and your palm going through downwards.

Relax your hand and curl your hands gently to make a fist. Squeeze you hands into a tight fist and maintain this gentle squeezing pressure for five seconds. You need to experience a gentle pull.

Uncurl your arms and function your hand in order that it's miles straight away once more. Hold your hand and hands certainly directly for another 5 seconds

Next, preserve your hand immediately and bypass your thumb in order that your thumb and index finger form a mouth or claw form. Hold this function for 5 seconds.

Relax your hand truly and repeat this together along with your left hand.

Repeat those bodily sports 2-3 instances with each hand.

Exercise 12 – Finger Pull Exercise

This exercising within reason easy and doesn't require any particular equipment or device as you are the usage of your very private force in the direction of you different hand. Be certain to splendid pull once more your palms as a ways as is snug as it is able to be so clean to over stretch without realizing.

Good For: Strengthening and stretching your fingers

Hold your right hand inside the front of you together with your hand outstretched and your palm going thru upwards.

Take your left hand and draw close to the thumb in your proper hand with hands.

Keep your hand at once and organisation and pull your thumb returned lightly till you experience a subtle stretch. Hold for 5 seconds.

Repeat this 5-10 instances with each hand.

Exercise thirteen – Foam Ball workout

For this workout, you may need a small foam ball that fits neatly in the palm of your hand. This is a specifically nicely exercising for strengthening the muscle groups for your hand, wrist and forearm and releasing any stress surrounding the median nerve. Ideally this exercise need to be finished together along with your hand mendacity on a flat surface.

Good For: Increasing power within the wrists and hands.

Begin by means of the use of maintaining your proper hand in the front of you together with your palm going thru up.

Place a small foam ball inside the center of your palm and near your palms round it.

Squeeze the ball until you can feel a snug stretch.

Hold this stretch for five seconds and increase this to ten seconds even as you sense able to.

Release your hands and lighten up your hand.

Repeat this workout once after which pass onto your left hand.

Repeat this exercise 2 times to begin with after which pass onto 5 repetitions even as you experience succesful.

Chapter 6: Putty Amongst Your Thumb And Forefinger

Gently squeeze the putty some of the ones palms and maintain for five seconds.

Next squeeze the putty among your thumb and center finger and keep for 5 seconds.

Continue to squeeze the putty among your thumb and each of your unique hands.

You can repeat this workout with every hand up to a few instances.

Exercise 16 – Putty Scissor Exercise

For this exercising, as with the only above, you'll want your putty. This is specially proper for stopping pain within the fingers and stretching each the arms and wrist joints.

Good for: Finger Pain and numbness

Hold your hand within the the front of you, palm upwards and palms spread apart.

Place a small ball of putty among your thumb and forefinger and squeeze gently for five seconds. Then location it among your forefinger and index finger and squeeze lightly. Repeat this technique till you have got were given reached your little finger.

Repeat up to 3 instances with each hand.

Exercise 17 – Finger Spread Putty Exercise

Again, as above, you will want a small ball of putty. If you are able to stretch the putty in the direction of this exercise even barely then keep in mind your self to have performed some issue. The idea isn't without a doubt to pull the putty an excessive amount of certainly so virtually make sure that you can experience your muscle corporations and hands stretching gently.

Good for: Flexing and strengthening the hands

Hold a small, flattened piece of putty on your left hand. Position your right hand in order that the recommendations of your palms are squeezed collectively.

Place the small, flattened piece of putty on top of your arms and try to spread the putty aside using the guidelines of your palms.

Repeat this together with your super hand.

Exercise 18 – Pencil finger extension

This exercising is exceptional for growing strength inside the fingers and wrist joints. The pencil is excellent because it offers you a few factor to capture onto due to this that your muscle mass are constantly working in the course of the exercising.

Good For: Keeping the fingers and wrists flexible

Hold your hand in front of you and maintain a pencil among your arms so you are forming a small fist with the pencil in between your arms.

Grip the pencil and preserve it among your palms with a touch pressure.

Bend your hand to and fro gently spherical five times.

Continue to grip the pencil and maintain your hand in the the the front of you all once more together together with your arm stretched out.

Gently fold your hand inwards, toward your palm as far as you can. Hold for 10 seconds.

Return your hand to its ordinary characteristic after which bend your wrist backwards as a long way as is snug, despite the fact that gripping the pencil.

Exercise 19 – Advanced Weight Wrist Flex Exercise

Good for: Strengthening the wrists, arms and palms

This exercising is designed to enhance the energy in your fingers and wrists with the aid of way of manner of the utilization of every an workout or home made weight (e.G. A tin of beans). This shape of weight is especially top for strengthening the wrist muscles and decreasing pressure on the nerves within the hand. In time you need to boom power and it'll in all likelihood reduce signs and symptoms of carpal tunnel syndrome pretty considerably.

Note: this workout can be too strenuous if you've simplest definitely said to exercising your wrist, hands and hands so it's far an concept to head away this workout until you feel capable to complete some bodily sports in your own with out causing your self any pain or pain.

Begin thru the usage of keeping your hand inside the front of you with a light weight or a tin of beans on your hand.

Stretch your arm out collectively along with your palm down and slowly bend your wrist upwards.

Continue to stretch your wrist as a protracted manner as feels snug.

Hold this stretch for 10 seconds.

Return your wrist to its ordinary function.

Then gently stretch your wrist down, preserve for 10 seconds and lighten up your wrist.

Repeat this five-10 times with every hand.

Exercise 20 – Gentle Neck Exercise

This exercise is superb for stretching the neck and pinnacle arm and therefore freeing tension surrounding the median nerve. If you be afflicted by any ache or specific symptoms for your decrease or top arm then this exercising is a great concept to try.

Good For: Relieving anxiety and pain in the arm

Stand upright along side your fingers by way of the use of your components.

Shrug your shoulders up, within the path of the sky and keep for five seconds.

Release all anxiety to your shoulders for 5 seconds after which squeeze them all over again so you create a shrugging movement.

Next, squeeze your shoulders lower back so that you are pinching your shoulder blades as close to collectively as possible. You should enjoy a moderate tug but no pain at this element

Hold this for 10 seconds.

As quick as you've finished maintaining the preceding feature, shrug your shoulders forwards this time so that you are spacing your shoulder blades aside.

Stop at the same time as you feel a slight tug and hold for every different 10 seconds.

Relax this characteristic and repeat 3-five times.

Other forms of remedy – Alternative Treatments

There are many opportunity treatments to pick from in case you are affected by the signs and symptoms and symptoms of RSI or Carpal Tunnel Syndrome. For a few human beings, opportunity remedies paintings to a degree and relieve their signs at the equal time as for others, possibility cures don't have any effect the least bit. Usually, those type of treatments aren't appeared thru manner of the medical profession as being specifically helpful and feature usually not been installed to work as human research and research in the ones areas are lacking.

However, if you are struggling to relieve your signs and symptoms thru traditional medication and need to avoid surgical treatment, there may be no motive why specific sorts of treatment cannot assist. Below you may discover a listing of the most famous alternative treatments and remedies.

Yoga

Some acquire as real with that yoga lets in to every save you and relieve the signs and symptoms and symptoms of carpal tunnel syndrome. There is confined evidence to enables the blessings of yoga for treating CTS however it is substantially diagnosed that yoga stretches and strengthens the joints. Therefore, in idea, yoga carrying activities that in particular recognition at the arms, wrists and fingers may additionally have some effect in relieving strain at the median nerve.

There are numerous one-of-a-type yoga physical video video games and a few practitioners have advanced new techniques and physical video games for alleviating the signs and symptoms of Carpal tunnel syndrome. If you're inquisitive about trying yoga then make sure to carry out a touch research, appearance on-line for brought records after which find out a licensed practitioner.

Acupuncture

Acupuncture is a well-known possibility remedy for treating Carpal tunnel Syndrome although it has not but been mounted to paintings as research is constrained in the region of possibility remedies and CTS.

Acupuncture for carpal tunnel syndrome works with the aid of way of placing skinny needles into areas in the forearm wrist, hand, thumb and arms. It works thru boosting the frame's natural pain relieving chemicals and anti inflammatory residences. It is concept to restore everyday nerve characteristic over time similarly to relieving ache in the quick term.

Chiropractic Therapies

It is idea that some chiropractic techniques can help to lessen the ache related to carpal tunnel syndrome in addition to decreasing stress surrounding the median nerve, however the truth that this has now not but been installation. Generally, chiropractic strategies range but most practitioners aim to launch anxiety with the aid of manipulating the upper and lower palms, wrists and hands. Mostly, chiropractic strategies are pretty easy and include a mixture of rubdown and manipulation of the bones and muscle tissue so that you can provide remedy of symptoms and symptoms.

Sufferers of CTS who've benefited from journeying a chiropractor have stated accelerated electricity and movement within the wrists, fingers and hands on the facet of a first-rate deal an awful lot less ache.

Ice Packs & Heat packs

Ice and heat packs are a very quick-time period choice to the ache because of carpal tunnel syndrome and they are every so often encouraged by means of scientific doctors and medical practitioners for immediate, quick term treatment so that you can keep with what you propose to do. If you are tormented by immoderate infection or throbbing or stabbing pains then an ice p.C. Can be a top notch concept.

Ideally, you ought to wrap a small ice % in a thin towel and region it over your hand, wrist or some thing location is most painful for 10 mins.

Heat packs also are a splendid concept for lowering pain and they're a really perfect brief term answer. If you aren't suffering from irritation then a warm temperature % is probably higher than an ice p.C. As it's far greater soothing and combats pain better than ice.

To prevent ache with warm temperature you can soak your arms in warmness or warm water for 10 – 20 mins each time you revel in it's far essential; this works well in advance than bed because it soothes the muscle organizations. You additionally can purchase mainly designed heat pads and packs from close by chemists or shops without the want for a prescription. Apply those to the affected location following the instructions for not than 20 minutes.

Sports tape

Sports tape is typically utilized by athletes, sports activities activities sports fans and physiotherapists so you can preserve the muscular tissues in a unmarried vicinity and keep away from any greater stress being located at the affected region. Sports tape isn't some aspect that is usually used for Carpal Tunnel Syndrome however it could function an alternative for a wrist splint, that would regularly get in the manner whilst searching for to carry out everyday responsibilities.

You should buy sports activities sports tape quite a first rate deal anywhere in recent times and you can generally locate it both online or in shops. As a large guiding principle you need to place the tape in order that it allows and covers your wrist and fingers even though there are various unique techniques of taping your wrist that allows you to offer resource for CTS.

If you would like to analyze greater approximately a way to tape your wrist so that it relieves ache and gives help, take a look on-line in which you'll locate masses of records and suggestions.

Vitamin B6

Vitamin B6 has been positioned to be related to carpal tunnel syndrome in numerous precise research studies. The principle is that each low tiers or a deficiency in nutrition B6 will increase in place of motives the symptoms of carpal tunnel syndrome Research has determined that low levels of Vitamin b6 increase the frequency and severity of CTS symptoms.

You should buy nutrients B6 capsules from health stores and over-the-counter in chemists however in advance than taking any more dietary supplements, it's far typically surely beneficial to test at the side of your medical doctor or clinical practitioner first. If you're reluctant to take vitamins tablets then you can constantly up your intake of this unique weight-reduction plan through your weight loss plan.

Foods which consist of sweet potatoes, salmon, turkey, and bananas all contain Vitamin B6 so if you need to increase your consumption of B6, it's miles crucial to attempt to embody the ones for your weight loss program wherein you can.

Arnica

Arnica is considered a homeopathic remedy that combats ache and sore muscle groups; those are really of the motives why it's miles this type of famous pain-reliever for CTS sufferers. Usually, arnica is available in a gel or cream shape and may be applied to the wrist, hand and forearm with the intention to lessen aches and pains.

Chapter 7: How To Diagnose Carpal Tunnel Syndrome

There are numerous steps worried within the evaluation of carpal tunnel syndrome, together with a bodily exam, imaging checks, and nerve feature exams. A individual's signs, that would encompass numbness, tingling, and weak spot in the palms and hands, can also lead a medical doctor to suspect carpal tunnel syndrome. The supplier will likewise get a few facts approximately the character's medical history, which consist of any hidden activities or drug remedies that is probably including to their element results.

The first step in diagnosing carpal tunnel syndrome is a physical examination. A healthcare expert will have a look at the patient's hand and finger power, flexibility, and sensitivity inside the route of this exam. The Tinel's sign or Phalen's take a look at, as an instance, can also be used to assess the median nerve's characteristic. To elicit a response from the median nerve, those assessments contain tapping the wrist or keeping the wrist in a flexed function for severa seconds.

Carpal tunnel syndrome also can be recognized with imaging checks. Any abnormalities inside the bones, tendons, or exceptional structures of the wrist and hand that can be contributing to the compression of the median nerve can be diagnosed with the help of X-rays, MRI scans, and ultrasounds. In addition, the ones exams can rule out special conditions that could have comparable symptoms and signs and symptoms and signs and symptoms, like nerve damage or arthritis.

Another crucial device for diagnosing carpal tunnel syndrome is nerve characteristic trying out. These assessments can help decide the amount and region of nerve damage by the use of manner of measuring the electric impulses sent by way of way of manner of the median nerve. Electromyography (EMG) and nerve conduction research (NCS) are not unusual nerve function assessments. Small electrodes are connected to a device that measures nerve feature in some unspecified time in the future of those assessments, which can be completed on the pores and skin.

The electrical interest of muscle mass throughout contraction and relaxation is measured with the useful resource of EMG. This test can also display screen nerve damage that motives reduced muscle hobby within the hand and wrist in people with carpal tunnel syndrome. NCS estimates the velocity at which electric signals journey via the nerves. This test may also moreover display slowed or decreased symptoms in the median nerve in human beings with carpal tunnel syndrome.

Carpal tunnel syndrome can occasionally be recognized with more exams. Blood checks can prevent hidden situations that might be along with to nerve harm, like thyroid problems or diabetes. A minimally invasive surgical treatment known as arthroscopy can help within the identity and treatment of any structural abnormalities within the wrist that may be ensuing in nerve compression.

A thorough evaluation of a person's signs and symptoms, clinical facts, physical examination, imaging, and nerve characteristic exams are all crucial for the prognosis of carpal tunnel syndrome.

Physical examination

A bodily exam is frequently carried out so that it will make a evaluation of carpal tunnel syndrome. A thorough clinical statistics and exam of the affected character's symptoms and signs and symptoms and symptoms generally precede the physical examination for carpal tunnel syndrome. The affected character is requested to offer an explanation for the sort of ache, how awful it's miles, how lengthy it lasts, and any activities that make the pain worse or higher. With this statistics, the medical physician can higher recognize the affected man or woman's scenario and devise the great remedy technique.

The clinical medical doctor tests for signs and symptoms and signs and symptoms of carpal tunnel syndrome at some point of a bodily examination after taking the affected character's clinical records. The evaluation often starts offevolved with the health practitioner comparing the affected man or woman's hand power and preserve. Asking the affected character to squeeze the scientific health practitioner's palms or keep a ball among their fingers accomplishes this.

Then, the medical health practitioner checks for the presence of swelling, contamination, or delicacy within the wrist and encompassing region. This is finished thru touching the location and surveying for suffering and delicacy. The health practitioner can also additionally moreover likewise check for muscle decay or shortcoming through surveying the patient's thumb, pointer, and center finger energy.

The Phalen's test, wherein the affected person's wrists are held in a flexed role for one minute to see if it reasons their signs and symptoms, can be completed thru the scientific health practitioner. Also common is the Tinel's sign test, in which the wrist is tapped to appearance if it reasons any ache or tingling in the fingers.

In some instances, the clinical clinical physician may additionally verify the analysis with the useful resource of sporting out nerve conduction studies (NCS) or electromyography (EMG). NCS measures the charge at which nerve indicators journey through the wrist, even as EMG measures the electrical interest of muscle mass and nerves. These checks are not usually vital for a habitual assessment however is probably beneficial in complicated instances.

When the analysis of carpal tunnel syndrome is confirmed, treatment alternatives may be stated with the affected character. Splinting, medication, physical treatment, and, in immoderate instances, surgical treatment are all types of remedy. In order to keep away from long-time period complications like muscle atrophy or nerve harm, it's miles important to cope with this condition as short as viable.

A crucial step in the analysis of carpal tunnel syndrome is the bodily exam. By cautiously evaluating the patient's side outcomes and appearing one of a type checks, docs can distinguish the purpose for the affected individual's aggravation and recommend a turning into treatment. The affected person's nice of existence can be greater appropriate, and lengthy-time period headaches can be averted, through early evaluation and remedy of carpal tunnel syndrome.

Diagnostic tests

Managing signs and stopping the situation's improvement require prompt detection and diagnosis. The analysis of CTS can be confirmed through using some of diagnostic exams.

Some of the tests that may be used to diagnose carpal tunnel syndrome are as follows:

1. Tinel's Sign Test::

One of the oldest techniques for diagnosing CTS is the Tinel's Sign Test. The median nerve in the wrist can be tapped or lightly pressed for the easy test. The take a look at is deemed great if the affected person reports tingling, numbness, or electric powered powered-like shocks all of the manner all of the way down to the fingers in their hand.

The nerve inflammation this is the maximum not unusual purpose of CTS can be detected the usage of the Tinel's Sign Test.

2. Phalen's Test:

The Phalen's Test is some other test that analyzes CTS. Holding the fingers in a decrease again-to-decrease back position, bending the wrists at a ninety-degree attitude, and pressing the backs of the palms together are the components of the test.

If the affected man or woman encounters loss of life, shivering, or pain within the arms in somewhere spherical one second, the check is taken into consideration as fantastic. According to the test, CTS is added on through stress on the median nerve.

3. Electromyogram (EMG) and Nerve Conduction Study (NCS):

Although EMG and NCS are two notable tests, they'll be frequently finished concurrently to diagnose CTS. Recording the electric indicators which can be despatched with the aid of way of the muscle agencies and nerves is one of the checks.

The EMG take a look at statistics muscle movement, on the equal time as the NCS continues the electric movement inside the nerves. To stimulate the median nerve, a healthcare expert also can additionally insert a small electrode into the affected individual's hand. The take a look at estimates the nerve's reaction time and what type of electric powered float is communicated through the nerve.

The analysis of CTS is confirmed if the test reveals a prolonged reaction time or low levels of electrical present day-day transmitted via the median nerve.

four. Ultrasonography:

Another non-invasive approach for diagnosing CTS is ultrasonography. The check uses immoderate-recurrence sound waves to make a photo of the middle nerve in the wrist. The check permits find out any changes within the shape of the nerve and measures the thickness of the nerve.

Pregnant girls, who may additionally moreover revel in swelling and elevated pressure at the median nerve, are specially genuine applicants for ultrasonography for the detection of CTS.

5. Magnetic Resonance Imaging (MRI):

Using radio waves and magnetic fields, an MRI is a greater advanced test that produces photos of the median nerve and the tissues that surround it.

Chapter 8: Rest And Splinting

Giving the affected hand and wrist enough relaxation is one of the handiest remedies for carpal tunnel syndrome. The strain positioned on the median nerve is lessened via way of rest, which permits reduce the swelling and infection inside the place. Besides, relaxation likewise assists with lightening the aggravation related to carpal passage sickness, providing you with some without a doubt essential consolation.

With regards to resting the impacted hand and wrist, bracing is the high-quality approach. A resource is a device that holds the wrist and hand in a nonpartisan role, preserving the tension off the middle nerve. Wearing a brace assists with immobilizing the wrist, reducing the hazard of extra damage, and permitting it to rest. This reduces ache, numbness, and tingling, allowing you to perform everyday activities with out making your signs and symptoms and signs and symptoms worse.

There are a few types of braces that can be applied for carpal tunnel syndrome. The wrist splint is one of the maximum not unusual styles of splints. Splints for the wrist are available in masses of sizes and are fabricated from sturdy substances like metal or plastic. The brace suits over the wrist and covers the palm and the rear of the hand, preserving it immobilized.

One more form of assist that is possible for carpal tunnel disorder is the night time time brace. Most of the time, night time time splints are worn at night to keep the hand and wrist in a independent function at the identical time as you sleep. In evaluation to wrist splints, they may be manufactured from soft substances and are more cushty to position on for prolonged durations of time. By wearing a night brace, you could partake in a tranquil night time time's rest with out being dissatisfied via the torment and uneasiness delivered about by the usage of carpal tunnel syndrome.

Rest and splinting have to move hand in hand if you want to effectively manage carpal tunnel syndrome. Rest and bracing artwork collectively at the hip to decrease the tension on the middle nerve and reduce the aggravation and inconvenience added approximately through the scenario. However, you ought to make sure that you are using the best splint within the proper way.

For the extremely good in shape and shape of splint, you need to communicate for your medical doctor earlier than shopping one. Your physician will test your symptoms and signs and symptoms and symptoms and inform you which ones ones splint is excellent for dealing with them. You want to ensure that you are wearing the splint correctly as quickly as you've got it.

Physical Therapy and Occupational Therapy

Physical treatment is a notable manner to deal with carpal tunnel syndrome as it lets in make more potent the muscle tissue within the hand and forearm and reduces symptoms and symptoms.

Exercise-based healing for carpal passage infection is a essential piece of treatment for this circumstance. You will collect assist from a bodily therapist in performing a whole lot of wearing activities which might be meant to reinforce the muscular tissues for your hand and forearm and alleviate carpal tunnel syndrome signs and signs and signs. In bodily remedy for carpal tunnel syndrome, a number of the simplest physical video games are as follows:

1. Wrist Flexion and Extension Exercises designed to decorate the muscles inside the forearm that control the wrist joint include wrist flexion and extension carrying activities. The wrist joint is moved via some of movement in the ones sports activities, which permits to enhance electricity and flexibility. Simply skip your wrist up and down at the equal time as preserving a moderate weight in your hand to perform wrist flexion and extension sports activities.

2. Finger Stretching Exercises

Exercises for stretching the fingers are speculated to make the muscle agencies in the fingers and palms extra bendy and strong. In those physical activities, you hold your hand out in the the front of you, stretch your hands as some distance as they may be capable of pass, after which maintain that feature for some seconds in advance than freeing it.

3. Grip Strengthening Exercises Grip-strengthening wearing sports purpose to bolster the muscular tissues in the forearm and hand that grip gadgets. To make stronger your grip, you use a hand gripper or a resistance band in those carrying events.

4. Range of Motion Exercises

These are bodily video games for Increasing the potential and energy of the muscular tissues inside the hand and forearm with fashion of muscle companies movement. These sports include shifting the hand and wrist thru pretty various motion, like growing a clench hand and then turning in it.

five. Nerve Gliding Exercises

Nerve gliding sports sports are designed to stretch the median nerve and alleviate carpal tunnel syndrome signs and symptoms. The motive of those carrying sports, which may be designed to stretch the median nerve, is to transport the hand and wrist in particular styles.

Physical remedy is a splendid approach for treating carpal passage sickness, as it assists with reinforcing the muscular tissues inside the hand and decrease arm and mitigates the component effects of this situation. As well as gambling out the sports activities sports portrayed over, an real professional will likewise assist you with distinguishing any bodily games or propensities that might be inclusive of on your thing outcomes, like composing or associated with a mouse for extended time frames. You can control your carpal tunnel syndrome greater successfully and beautify your famous fantastic of life thru strolling with a bodily therapist.

A vital part of treating carpal tunnel syndrome is occupational treatment. It desires to alleviate carpal tunnel syndrome symptoms and signs at the same time as concurrently enhancing a affected man or woman's capability to engage in paintings, pursuits, and every day sports. The important goal of phrase-associated remedy is to reestablish the affected individual's wrist, hand, and finger portability and functionality through restorative sports and ergonomic changes.

Therapeutic physical sports

Therapeutic wearing occasions are one of the high-quality remedies for carpal tunnel syndrome. Word-associated experts are proficient at making customized exercising packages which might be tailored to every affected person's particular requirements and capacities. Some of these wearing activities might be:

1. Wrist flexion and extension: The wrist is flexed and prolonged towards resistance, together with a rubber band, in this

workout. It enables to reduce the stress on the median nerve thru strengthening the muscles in the wrist.

2. Fingers and thumbs competition : Touching the thumb with each finger sequentially is the reason of this workout. It increases the electricity and dexterity of the arms and thumbs, which might also additionally lessen the impact at the median nerve and wrist.

three. Middle nerve glides: The median nerve in the wrist is lightly moved from side to side inside the path of this exercising. It aids in enhancing nerve mobility and lowering nerve compression.

4. Strengthening the grip: Squeezing a ball or putty improves grip electricity on this exercise. It can likewise assist with lessening the burden at the wrist and center nerve.

Benefits of occupational remedy

Occupational remedy is a treatment alternative for carpal tunnel syndrome that doesn't incorporate surgical remedy or tablets. It can lessen pain and distinct symptoms and signs on the identical time as also enhancing a affected man or woman's wrist, hand, and finger mobility and feature. Occupational remedy can also help sufferers in resuming their commonplace paintings, pastimes, and each day sports activities on the identical time as keeping their independence.

The use of occupational remedy as a treatment choice for carpal tunnel syndrome has been mounted thru studies.

Nonsteroidal Anti-inflammatory Drugs (NSAIDs)

Nonsteroidal Anti-Inflammatory tablets (NSAIDs) are a preferred magnificence of prescriptions used to lessen ache, contamination, and swelling in first-rate illnesses. Carpal tunnel syndrome (CTS) is the form of situations. In the treatment of carpal tunnel syndrome sufferers' ache and contamination, nonsteroidal anti inflammatory drugs (NSAIDs) had been validated to be powerful.

Depending at the severity of the scenario, there are masses of remedy options for carpal tunnel syndrome. Moderate treatment draws close to; for example, wrist guide and exercising-based healing are generally the primary traces of guard for patients with mild to direct carpal passage situations. Notwithstanding, patients with greater intense facet results can also require greater forceful treatment, which incorporates NSAIDs, scientific strategies, or a mixture of each.

For an entire lot of medical situations, which includes carpal tunnel syndrome, nonsteroidal anti inflammatory tablets (NSAIDs) are regularly prescribed.

Prostaglandins, the chemical substances in the body that motive pain and infection, are inhibited through the ones medicinal pills. By lessening the ranges of prostaglandins within the body, NSAIDs can successfully decrease pain and aggravation in sufferers with carpal tunnel syndrome.

The maximum broadly diagnosed styles of NSAIDs applied in the manage of carpal passage contamination are ibuprofen, headache medicine, and naproxen. These pills are to be had with out a prescription and are fairly secure for brief use. However, patients want to be aware about the possibility of unfavorable results including ulcers within the stomach, gastrointestinal bleeding, and damage to the liver and kidneys. Before taking NSAIDs, sufferers who already have situations like excessive blood strain or coronary coronary heart sickness ought to talk to their medical medical doctor.

The severity of the situation determines how effectively NSAIDs treat carpal tunnel syndrome. NSAIDs can extensively reduce pain and decorate hand functionality in patients with mild to slight symptoms. However, NSAIDs won't be sufficient for sufferers with more extreme signs, necessitating extra aggressive remedy alternatives like surgical procedure.

Other remedies for carpal tunnel syndrome, including wrist splinting and bodily treatment, additionally may be blended with NSAIDs. Carpal tunnel syndrome signs can be alleviated most correctly with a mixture of remedies in a few times.

Patients with carpal tunnel syndrome can gain from NSAIDs as a remedy choice. In sufferers with moderate to mild signs, those pills can efficiently reduce pain and infection. However, more aggressive remedy, which includes surgical operation, may be required for patients with more excessive signs and symptoms and signs.

Steroid Injections

Steroid injections are a common remedy preference. Corticosteroids are applied in steroid injections to lessen infection, ease pain and ache, and enhance nerve function.

Steroid injections were demonstrated to be very powerful in treating CTS, especially in the early ranges. Utilizing a small needle, the steroid is injected without delay into the affected location. This can be executed in an outpatient clinic or clinical place of business. Patients are usually capable of resume their ordinary sports right away following the injection, and it's far commonly safe.

Steroid injections have a quite brief onset of movement, because of this they alleviate ache fast. This is a significant advantage. Typically, the injection reduces infection by using suppressing the immune device's reaction. Due to their anti-inflammatory houses, corticosteroids useful resource in relieving contamination-related signs. When infused, the corticosteroid makes a enjoy thru the flow into system to the kindled vicinity, wherein it's going to paintings swiftly to provide assist.

Steroid injections have a high fulfillment fee for treating CTS, however there are some feasible element results. Normal aftereffects might also moreover embody short deadness, shivering, and contamination at the infusion website. In unusual times, bleeding or contamination might also get up on the website online. However, those uncommon risks mild in evaluation to the advantages of steroid injections.

Pain, numbness, and tingling in the arms, wrists, and fingers because of CTS can appreciably have an impact on someone's each day sports activities. Steroid infusions are a valuable remedy preference which can help with lessening contamination, decreasing torment and inconvenience, and reestablishing nerve capability. It is a remedy desire this is mainly short and stable, with minor side effects which is probably clean to control. To decorate their excellent of lifestyles, sufferers with symptoms of CTS must are searching out scientific interest as quickly as viable and test out numerous remedy options, which incorporates steroid injections.

Open Surgery

There are numerous methods to this problem; be that as it is able to, an energetically recommended approach is the Carpal Tunnel Surgical Procedure. In this method, a professional makes a touch cut within the center of the hand to allow the anxiety out of the middle nerve. Patients can commonly go back to their houses the identical day, and this approach normally takes one or hours. Carpal tunnel syndrome can be dealt with with surgical procedure, but patients ought to moreover speak to their doctors and test out other alternatives.

At the factor while all of us chooses to have a carpal tunnel clinical technique, they need to to start with set themselves up every intellectually and in fact. Choosing a expert and expert health care professional is the maximum crucial step in training. Patients need to meet with the scientific expert to ensure they're cushty and confident in their capabilities in advance than you decide.

The patient ought to additionally find out approximately the way themselves. Before gift system any surgery, it's miles vital to be privy to the capability effects as well as the functionality thing consequences. One technique for training your self the carpal passage clinical approach is through way of travelling a reliable scientific services website or speakme with any person who has lengthy long gone via the medical machine.

It is time to begin pre-surgical treatment arrangements once the affected man or woman has selected a certified scientific health practitioner and is cushty with the manner. Most of the time, the medical doctor will can help you understand to make some modifications on your manner of existence that will help you manipulate your symptoms and signs and symptoms and get equipped for the surgery. Patients might be encouraged to carry out specific hand and wrist bodily sports, restrict in reality difficult art work, or attempt not to involve the impacted hand as masses as can also need to pretty be predicted. At instances, sufferers might be approached to take specific nutrients or tablets to help their today's well-being in advance than medical approaches.

Patients will gain fashionable anesthesia the day of the surgery. During the approach, this type of anesthesia makes the affected character unconscious, just so they won't experience any ache or soreness. The scientific tool itself includes the expert making a chunk get admission to point in the middle of the hand, after which they may tenderly stretch or lessen the tendons and tissues in the carpal passage to ease strain from the middle nerve. In a few times, any infected or damaged nerve or tissue that is inflicting the trouble can be eliminated through manner of the usage of the healthcare expert.

After the surgical treatment is completed, the doctor will carefully near the incision and cowl the hand with a protective bandage. The majority of patients are able to pass again to their normal activities the equal day as their surgical treatment, but they may need a while to get higher.

Patients are suggested to clean and dry their arms on the surgical web web page at the same time as they're getting better.

Chapter 9: Acupuncture

While there are some traditional drugs for carpal tunnel conditions, consisting of meds, exercising-based totally definitely healing, and medical strategies, a rising type of people are going to acupuncture remedy for help. Acupuncture remedy is an vintage Chinese exercising that includes the addition of slight needles to precise regions of the frame. It is idea that this remedy can beautify circulate, lessen contamination, and alleviate ache with the useful resource of way of stimulating the frame's herbal recovery capabilities.

As a non-invasive, safe treatment preference for carpal tunnel syndrome, acupuncture is gaining reputation. The benefits of acupuncture for carpal tunnel syndrome, the science at the back of its efficacy, and what to anticipate in the route of an acupuncture consultation will all be said in this article.

Acupuncture's Positive Effects on Carpal Tunnel Syndrome Acupuncture has a number of splendid consequences on carpal tunnel syndrome, together with the subsequent:

1. Relief from soreness: Needle therapy is idea for its aggravation-alleviating affects, making it a high-quality remedy for carpal tunnel syndrome. Acupuncture has been examined in studies to reduce ache and ache with the aid of manner of stimulating the frame's herbal production of endorphins.

2. Diminishes Aggravation: By developing the flow of blood and oxygen to the affected area, acupuncture can help in decreasing infection within the hand and wrist. Since contamination is one of the critical reasons of carpal tunnel syndrome, lowering irritation could make signs and symptoms lots better.

three. Further develops nerve functionality: tingling, numbness, and weak spot can be reduced thru improved nerve feature in the wrist and hand through acupuncture. Acupuncture can assist in reversing nerve damage due to carpal tunnel syndrome thru using stimulating nerve regeneration.

4. Non-invasive: Acupuncture is a non-invasive remedy without a factor outcomes, now not like treatment or surgical treatment. As a result, it's miles a greater stable choice for those who determine on not to take treatment or undergo invasive techniques.

The technology inside the again of acupuncture remedy for carpal tunnel syndromes

While the additives inside the returned of needle remedy are not completely understood, a few studies have researched the viability of needle treatment for carpal tunnel syndrome.

A systematic take a look at that end up published inside the Journal of Orthopedic Surgery and Research decided that acupuncture helped carpal tunnel syndrome sufferers enjoy lots much less pain and function better. According to a excellent test that emerge as published inside the Journal of Alternative and Complementary Medicine, acupuncture became virtually as effective as splinting at assuaging carpal tunnel syndrome symptoms and symptoms.

It is idea that acupuncture works with the beneficial resource of stimulating the release of neurotransmitters that manage ache and temper, like serotonin and norepinephrine.

Yoga and Stretching Exercises

As we spend extra time typing, texting, and the usage of handheld devices, CTS has come to be a commonplace hassle in the virtual age. Yoga and stretching physical video games, but, can assist alleviate CTS signs and symptoms and hold them from going on again.

Let's have a look at numerous yoga stretches and poses that alleviate CTS symptoms.

1. Wrist circles

This clean workout enables relieve pressure on the median nerve inside the wrist. Make fine your fingers are pointing within the course of the ceiling as you start through extending your arm at once in front of you. Presently, step by step turn your wrist in a roundabout movement, first clockwise and later on adversarial to clockwise. In each path, repeat this ten to 15 instances.

2. Cow face pose

The cow face pose stretches the wrists, arms, and forearm muscle groups. Start with the aid of using sitting leg-over-leg at the ground along side your fingers within the lower back of your decrease decrease back. Over your shoulder and closer to the center of your lower once more, deliver your right hand up. Try to clasp your hands collectively together along with your left hand as you beautify it up in the route of your shoulder blade. You can hold onto a towel if you are unable to clasp your arms.

3. Prayer pose: This pose lets in to make the wrist more bendy and mobile. Begin through the use of sitting inside the again of you at the side of your palms squeezed together earlier than your chest. Gradually decrease your elbows in the direction of the floor, keeping your fingers collectively. Stand employer on this foothold for 10–15 seconds, and in a while discharge.

four. Eagle fingers

This posture extends the shoulders and the pinnacle another time muscles, that would alleviate strain within the wrists. Stand right now collectively along side your arms at your components to start. Cross your right arm over your left as you deliver your palms in the front of your chest. Bring your palms collectively in order that they're touching. Bend your elbows. Lift your elbows towards the roof and stand enterprise on this footing for 30 seconds. Rehash on the opportunity side.

5. Downward dog pose

The downward dog pose stretches the whole body, stretching the palms and wrists. Start on all fours along with your arms at the ground and your knees bent. Straighten your legs and arms as you slowly boom your hips toward the ceiling. Keep your palms shoulder-width aside and your palms unfold out. Keep this feature for amongst 30 and 60 seconds.

6. Finger stretches

Stretching the arms is an exercising that works on the muscle tissue inside the palms and may help with CTS signs and symptoms and signs and symptoms. With your palm going through down, increase your arm in the front of you to begin. Utilize your one-of-a-type hand to tenderly draw your palms lower again inside the path of your wrist, preserving each finger for 10–15 seconds.

Chiropractic Manipulation

Manual treatment strategies are utilized in chiropractic manipulation to adjust the frame's joints. The musculoskeletal system will regain normal feature, mobility may be extra, and ache and infection is probably reduced because of these changes. To deal with a huge range of musculoskeletal situations, chiropractors rent loads of strategies, which includes spinal changes, joint mobilization, tender tissue manipulation, and stretching.

By lowering contamination inside the wrist and surrounding tissues and relieving strain on the median nerve, chiropractic manipulation can correctly deal with CTS signs. To treat CTS, chiropractors may additionally additionally furthermore lease lots of guide strategies, which include mobilizing the wrist and making changes to the bones of the hand and fingers. The aim of those techniques is to get the wrist shifting and aligned commonly, as a manner to lessen stress at the median nerve and assist with signs and symptoms and signs and symptoms and symptoms.

Chiropractic manipulation can be a useful remedy for CTS, in line with a recent look at that have grow to be posted within the Journal of Manipulative and Physiological

Therapeutics. The evaluate accompanied a assembly of ninety one sufferers with gentle to direct CTS who got chiropractic manipulate inner a six-week time span. The research placed that sufferers encountered a big decrease in torment and improvement of their competencies following remedy. In addition, the look at decided that sufferers who obtained chiropractic care have been greater happy with their care than folks who obtained traditional health center remedy.

Even despite the fact that chiropractic manipulation can assist deal with CTS, now not all times of CTS are specific candidates for chiropractic care. In order to determine out what's inflicting your signs and whether or not chiropractic care is right for you, chiropractors will behavior an extensive examination. Chiropractic manipulation won't be the great remedy choice for you if you have accidents or first rate clinical conditions which might be causing your CTS symptoms and signs and symptoms.

If you decide to get CTS dealt with with chiropractic care, it's important to art work with an authorized chiropractor who is aware about the way to treat it. Based on your precise necessities and symptoms and signs, your chiropractor will behavior an in-intensity exam and create a custom designed remedy plan. Manual techniques, exercising remedy, and modifications for your way of existence, like making your place of business extra ergonomic, might also moreover all be part of the remedy.

Herbal Remedies and Supplements

As a herbal manner to govern their symptoms and signs, many people with carpal tunnel syndrome flip to herbal treatments and dietary supplements. Let's talk about some of the terrific dietary supplements and natural treatments for carpal tunnel syndrome.

1. Turmeric

Turmeric is a famous spice that has been utilized in ordinary Indian medicinal drug for quite some time. It has been tested that curcumin, a high-quality anti-inflammatory element, reduces ache and inflammation. Turmeric is accessible in outstanding bureaucracy, collectively with times, teas, and powders. Additionally, it may be used as a cooking spice. According to investigate, turmeric's capacity to lessen contamination and alleviate pain has been showed to be useful for humans with carpal tunnel syndrome.

2. Ginger

Ginger is a few other famous spice that has mitigating homes. Joint ache, arthritis, and special inflammatory situations are often treated with it. Ginger can be ate up in a whole lot of tactics, inclusive of drugs, ginger tea, smooth ginger root, and nutritional dietary dietary supplements. According to three studies, ginger may be beneficial for human beings with carpal tunnel syndrome due to its capacity to reduce contamination and alleviate ache.

3. Omega-three fatty acid

Omega-3 unsaturated fat are a shape of polyunsaturated fats this is located specifically kinds of fish, nuts, and seeds. They have been validated to reduce frame infection and characteristic anti inflammatory houses. Omega-three improvements are available in a single-of-a-kind systems, along with fish oil containers and krill oil times. Omega-3 dietary nutritional dietary supplements may be useful for humans with carpal tunnel syndrome, constant with some research, as they may help lessen contamination and ache.

4. Vitamin B6

Vitamin B6 The apprehensive system's proper operation is dependent on nutrients B6, a crucial nutrient. Neurotransmitters, which can be chemical substances that beneficial aid inside the transmission of signals amongst nerve cells, are produced thru it. Vitamin B6 dietary dietary supplements were confirmed in a few studies to help human beings with carpal tunnel syndrome with the useful resource of decreasing inflammation and improving nerve function.

Chapter 10: Ergonomics And Posture

In the age of innovation and superior correspondence, we frequently spend a long term slouched over a PC display display or composing away at our consoles. Unfortunately, an entire lot people don't recognize the results of our sedentary lifestyle till it's too past due. One of the maximum substantially recognized problems for folks that artwork prolonged hours is carpal tunnel syndrome (CTS).

Fortunately, simple ergonomic and posture strategies make it feasible to save you carpal tunnel syndrome. If you want to hold your fingers and wrists wholesome and reduce your chance of CTS, ergonomics and posture can skip a protracted manner. We'll take a look at a number of the strategies to prevent carpal tunnel syndrome through training ergonomics and retaining a wholesome posture.

The primary thing you have to recollect is your stance. When running, masses of people slouch or hunch in advance, in particular after they spend numerous time at a pc. CTS may be because of placing stress at the nerves and blood vessels to your neck, shoulder, hands, and fingers even as you are taking a seat in a horrible function. To prevent this, you actually need to sit down down down upright. Given that masses people spend limitless hours seated at our desks, that is a good deal less tough stated than performed. Be that as it may, it's crucial to cognizance on the way you're sitting and rise up, stretch, or walk round continuously.

A well-designed chair may want to make all the difference. Buy a chair with a seat and backrest that can be adjusted and right lumbar assist. You can regulate an adjustable chair to fit your table's height and guide well posture. Armrests need to additionally be protected on your chair so that you can type and not using a problem collectively along with your elbows resting on them and your shoulders last cushty.

The following level is to change your computer arrangement. Your laptop must be at eye stage, and each your keyboard and mouse must be on the equal degree and sincerely available. Because their mouse is simply too a ways faraway from them, many human beings with CTS need to again and again growth their arm. This is a few other difficulty that contributes to CTS and is referred to as repetitive pressure harm.

Furthermore, accurate typing is vital. Keep your wrists instantly as you kind by manner of positioning your keyboard in the the the front of you. Try not to wind your wrists or curve them at a point considering this comes down at the ligaments in your draw near. Assuming you study that you're experiencing issue keeping your wrists immediately, bear in thoughts using an ergonomic console or wrist facilitates. Support for the wrist assists you in retaining a without delay wrist and minimizing joint pressure.

Taking breaks is crucial. You need to take not unusual breaks in case you kind or work on the pc for hours. Your wrists and arms will have time to rest, stretch, and recover from the strain due to this. During the ones breaks, arise, walk spherical, or stretch your palms, palms, and shoulders.

Exercise and stretches

Carpal Tunnel Syndrome (CTS) has come to be a common state of affairs amongst human beings as we increasingly rely on generation and paintings extended hours at pc systems. The hand and wrist are suffering from this painful state of affairs, which moreover reasons tingling, numbness, and weak point. Be that as it could, with the right sports activities and stretches, preventing CTS is possible. The incredible physical sports and stretches for preventing carpal tunnel syndrome can be mentioned in this article.

1. Hand-extending Exercises

Hand-extending practices are the notable sports activities for preventing carpal tunnel syndrome. The following are more than one extending practices you can try:

Wrist flexor stretches.

Start with the useful useful resource of reputation instantly together with your toes shoulder-width aside to carry out this exercise. Stretch your arms directly out in advance than you, together along with your palms going thru every other. Now, together with your hands pointing

155

upward, lightly bend your wrist lower lower back within the route of you together along with your contrary hand. Repeat with the alternative hand after retaining this stretch for approximately 15–20 seconds.

Wrist extensor stretch

Start with the beneficial resource of popularity directly along side your ft shoulder-width apart to perform this workout. With your hands handling upward, boom your palms without delay out in the front of you. Now, gently bend your wrist toward the ground along side your palms pointing downward. Do this with the alternative hand. Repeat with the opposite hand after shielding this stretch for approximately 15–20 seconds.

Thumb stretchk:

Make a fist together at the side of your thumb indoors to start this exercising.

Now, circulate your thumb away from your palm with moderate strain till you experience a stretch on your thumb and the yet again of your hand. Repeat with the opportunity hand after protecting this stretch for about 15–20 seconds.

2. Grip Strengthening Exercises

By strengthening the hand and wrist, grip-strengthening bodily activities beneficial aid inside the prevention of carpal tunnel syndrome. Try a number of the wearing sports beneath.

Press Ball Exercise:

Hold a press ball or smooth ball for your palm to carry out this exercise. Release the ball after ten seconds of intense squeezing. Ten to fifteen times, do that exercising.

Hand gripper sports activities activities:

Hold a hand gripper in a single hand and squeeze it as tough as you could for ten seconds earlier than releasing to perform this exercise. With every hand, carry out this workout ten to 15 times.

Fingers physical video games:

To play out this interest, positioned your hand stage on a ground, then, at that detail, tap each finger independently as speedy as possible. Rehash this hobby for 30 seconds, then transfer palms and rehash.

three. Wrist Rotating Exercises

By improving wrist flexibility, wrist rotating physical sports beneficial useful resource in the prevention of carpal tunnel syndrome. Try a number of the carrying sports below.

Wrist Circles:

Start through using the usage of status at once collectively along with your feet shoulder-width aside to perform this exercise. For ten seconds, use your fingers to make small circles in a single direction earlier than switching to the opportunity.

Avoiding repetitive moves

Avoiding repetitive motions is one of the super methods to avoid carpal tunnel syndrome. This way delaying obligations that require a number of typing or writing. Take a spoil each hour to stretch your hands and wrists in case you kind lots at your computer, as an instance. Additionally, you could hire ergonomically designed device like a keyboard and mouse to relieve wrist and hand pressure.

One greater technique for stopping carpal passage is to exercising exceptional stance. Make sure your wrists are at once and your shoulders are snug at the same time as you're taking a seat down at a computer. Your wrists and arms will experience less strained due to this. To keep a impartial role to your wrists, you may additionally use a wrist relaxation.

Practice is furthermore huge for stopping carpal tunnel syndrome. Your palms and wrists may be strengthened via everyday workout, lowering your risk of developing carpal tunnel syndrome. There are many sports activities sports that you can do to reinforce your hands and wrists, for instance, wrist twists and finger expansions. You can also strive yoga or Pilates, which may be brilliant for making you more potent and more bendy everyday.

One greater technique for forestalling carpal passage ailment is to utilize the right approach whilst you're doing monotonous obligations. For example, at the same time as typing, take a look at to look that your palms are putting the keys with the best quantity of stress. On the off hazard which you are gambling an device, ensure you are keeping it because it ought to be and using the valid finger role.

Additionally, taking breaks for the duration of the day to relaxation your fingers and wrists is vital. In the occasion which you are composing or composing for a prolonged time frame, take some time without work like clockwork to increase your arms and wrists. Heat or bloodless remedy additionally can be used to reduce irritation and ache.

There are a few additional things you could do to keep away from carpal tunnel syndrome further to the ones hints. To keep your wrists in a impartial characteristic, as an instance, you may wear a brace or splint. You may additionally strive rubdown remedy or acupuncture, each of which could help reduce ache and infection.

In the occasion which you are encountering issue consequences of carpal passage sickness, it's far vital to look for remedy proper now. To alleviate your signs and symptoms, your scientific doctor may additionally additionally endorse bodily remedy, treatment, or surgical procedure. Your probabilities of having better from carpal tunnel syndrome are more appropriate if you are looking for for remedy as quick as feasible.

Carpal tunnel syndrome is a tough state of affairs that can be delivered about with the aid of redundant traits. Be that as it can, there are various topics you could do to save you carpal tunnel syndrome.

Workplace safety suggestions

Let's communicate about a few approaches that employees can keep away from carpal tunnel syndrome at artwork.

1. Your posture is one of the maximum critical factors to reflect onconsideration on whilst trying to prevent carpal tunnel syndrome. Unfortunate stance can location an unjustifiable burden in your muscle tissue, tendons, and nerves, making it nearly high quality that you'll come upon component effects of the carpal passage situation. You can lower your risk of growing this painful condition by way of using sitting up immediately, retaining your shoulders cushty, and standing instantly in place of bending over.

2. Take breaks. When you're running on initiatives that require you to apply your fingers and wrists masses, it's critical to take commonplace breaks. You may be able to unwind and stretch your fingers, hands, and wrists at the same time as

taking brief breaks, that could ease the stress to your muscular tissues and joints. While playing reprieves, it manner pretty a chunk to walk spherical and stretch your frame, consisting of your back, neck, and hands.

three. Stretch and schooling session usually.

Normal hobby and growing can help with similarly developing dissemination and flexibility, that could lower the hazard of carpal passage disease. Activities, for instance, hand and finger extensions, wrist twists, and shoulder rolls, may be finished in the course of breaks or while having some time off from composing at the console.

four. Utilize ergonomic machine. Employing ergonomic tool can useful aid in the prevention of carpal tunnel syndrome. Ergonomic consoles and mouse cushions are speculated to restriction the risk of wrist stress and assist you to artwork in a greater regular function. Other ergonomic hardware to keep in mind consists of movable seats and shows, in addition to ergonomic pens and pencils.

5. Take suitable relaxation.

It is critical to take great relaxation and get sufficient rest to save you carpal tunnel ailment. A sound night time time's sleep is crucial for first-rate fitness in giant, in conjunction with the health of the muscle mass, joints, and nerves. By causing muscle fatigue and tension, now not getting enough sleep have to make it much more likely that you may boom carpal tunnel syndrome.

6. Keep your fingers warmth.

Cold temperatures can demolish the aspect consequences of carpal tunnel syndrome, so it's far vital to keep your arms warmth. To keep your palms comfortable and decrease your chance of developing carpal tunnel syndrome, you may use hand heaters, gloves, or different gadgets that generate heat.

7. You want to are looking for scientific interest as soon as you have got a observe any signs and symptoms and signs of carpal tunnel syndrome, in conjunction with pain, numbness, or tingling on your arms, wrists, or fingers. The state of affairs may be better controlled with early analysis and remedy, and the sooner you are looking for for treatment, the higher your possibilities of achievement.

Healthy way of lifestyles choices

Maintaining real posture and ergonomics is one of the most important way of life options for stopping carpal tunnel syndrome. Maintaining a unbiased spine feature, which can lessen pressure for your palms and wrists, is made much less tough with top posture. It is essential to ensure that your chair is adjusted to the appropriate top and that the armrests aid your arms at the same time as operating at a computer. Moreover, a console and mouse which is probably at the proper level can reduce weight on all fours. If you discern with gadget or tool, check to appearance that they may be made to fit your body in an ergonomic way.

Carpal tunnel syndrome prevention can also advantage from stretching and exercise. The possibility of growing CTS can be reduced by way of developing wrist and hand flexibility through stretching physical sports. Wrist stretches and rotations, smooth bodily video video games, can help keep your wrist flexible. Customary hobby can likewise assist with in addition developing dissemination and lowering aggravation, that could make a contribution to the improvement of CTS.

Keeping a wholesome weight is a few different vital lifestyle choice that could assist prevent carpal tunnel syndrome. Being overweight can placed more strain to your joints, that might make you much more likely to get CTS. You can lower your chance of growing carpal tunnel syndrome and precise joint-related situations by way of ingesting a healthful diet regime and exercising frequently.

It is crucial to take not unusual breaks and avoid doing matters over and over over again that positioned stress for your wrists and hands. Take common breaks to stretch your wrists and circulate spherical if you kind or artwork at a computer for long periods of time. When lifting heavy gadgets or running with hand tool, don't use too much strain or grip. Also, don't keep your wrist in the same characteristic for too prolonged because of the reality doing so can positioned more strain on the median nerve.

Various way of life alternatives can aid within the prevention of carpal tunnel syndrome. You can reduce your chance of developing CTS with the useful resource of running in the direction of ergonomics and suitable posture, stretching, exercise, preserving a healthy weight, and taking commonplace breaks. You can help shield your hands and wrists and maintain correct ordinary fitness and health thru incorporating those wholesome manner of existence options into your every day routine.

How to avoid future flare-americaand save you re-damage

While CTS can't be cured, there are some subjects you can do to avoid flare-americaand re-harm. To avoid developing

CTS signs and symptoms in the destiny, try the following:

1. Practicing ergonomics and posture correctly is one of the essential elements that make a contribution to CTS. Sitting for huge stretches of time collectively with your wrist in a twisted or flexed characteristic can reason exorbitant tension at the center nerve, prompting the aspect consequences of CTS. When strolling along side your fingers for prolonged stretches of time, it's specially critical to preserve your posture and ergonomics in take a look at.

Keep your shoulders down, your elbows close to your frame, and your wrists in a unbiased function for proper posture. Adjust your computer and chair just so your fingers and wrists are in the right alignment together with your keyboard and mouse.

2. Regular stretching and exercise will allow you to save you CTS flare-u.S.A.With the useful resource of developing your flexibility and blood go along with the flow. Yoga and exclusive low-impact sports activities are specifically beneficial because of the truth they help you loosen up and relieve wrist anxiety.

Extending sports, for example, wrist flexion and augmentation, finger and thumb stretches, and lower arm stretches, can help with further developing your wrist versatility and reduce the hazard of CTS aspect results. Try to revel in reprieves from dreary sporting sports and stretch your hands and wrists normally.

three. When lifting and wearing heavy items, use the right strategies. Heavy lifting and sporting can positioned quite a few strain in your fingers and wrists, which could make you more likely to get CTS signs and symptoms and signs and symptoms and signs and symptoms and symptoms. Use right lifting and carrying strategies, which includes lifting together with your legs and retaining your wrists at once, to keep away from destiny flare-ups.

Use a strap or cope with to flippantly distribute the load of heavy devices whilst sporting them. Gripping subjects too tightly can exacerbate CTS signs and symptoms and symptoms as well.

four. Utilize a wrist splint or brace

In the occasion that you have encountered CTS aspect outcomes earlier than, wearing a wrist guide can assist with forestalling destiny eruptions. By preserving your wrist in a impartial function and imparting assist, a wrist splint can alleviate pressure to your median nerve.

Chapter 11: Coping With Ache

Perhaps the earliest issue that you could do is change your ordinary physical sports. It is important to keep away from or lower certain sports if you find out that they may be making your symptoms worse. This need to propose converting your artwork area or making use of precise hardware that is supposed to decrease the weight for your wrists.

One extra possible method for overseeing carpal passage sickness is to utilize facilitates. These are made specially to help the wrists and alleviate pain and pain. There are many precise types of braces, so you have to talk in your clinical doctor or bodily therapist about which one could be first-rate for you.

Naturally, preventing carpal tunnel syndrome from taking location inside the first region is the most green approach of handling it. This approach being attentive to how you operate your hands and wrists. For example, stretching your wrists and taking breaks can help prevent carpal tunnel syndrome.

However, no matter the exceptional preventative measures in place, carpal tunnel syndrome can still occur. Also, at the same time as that happens, there are some unique methodologies that may be a success.

Heat or cold therapy is one manner to alleviate ache and decrease contamination. Depending to your symptoms and signs, this can include using an ice % or a heating pad.

The use of rubdown remedy is but each different effective technique. This can ease ache and pain through easing muscle tension and developing blood go together with the go with the flow to the affected location.

Carpal tunnel syndrome may be treated with a large range of over-the-counter and pharmaceuticals. These might also want to contain calming medicinal drugs, pain relievers, or unique forms of drugs.

In the give up, there may be no "magic bullet" for treating carpal tunnel syndrome. However, it's far feasible to manipulate the circumstance's pain and ache with the beneficial useful resource of adopting a complete technique that includes pretty a few high-quality procedures.

Talking in your medical medical doctor or physical therapist about the diverse techniques that could paintings first-rate for you is critical if you have carpal tunnel syndrome. There are a whole lot of techniques that might help you in dealing with the ache of carpal tunnel syndrome and retaining a immoderate awesome of existence. Some of those strategies encompass altering your each day normal, utilising specialised machine, or studying possibility remedies like massage or medicine.

Managing every day sports

Living with carpal tunnel syndrome may be hard, specially in phrases of organizing one's day. Fortunately, you could manage the signs and symptoms of carpal tunnel syndrome and stay a more cushty lifestyles by way of using making a few simple changes for your ordinary. With carpal tunnel syndrome, it could be tough to keep up with normal activities.

1. Avoid repetitive sports. Repetitive sports activities activities like typing, stitching, and playing an tool are all most important individuals to carpal tunnel syndrome. Avoiding or minimizing those sports is essential if you want to lower your hazard of developing the state of

affairs or making the signs and signs and signs worse.

If your process calls that allows you to delivery your hands and wrists plenty, try to take common breaks and stretch. If you want to assist lessen the strain for your wrist, you have to recollect the usage of ergonomic tools and device like a wrist brace.

2. Keep your palms heat. Keeping your hands warmth can help with reducing firmness and uneasiness in the wrist and fingers. You can appoint hand warmers, gloves, or basically soak up your fingers in heat water for more than one moments to facilitate the aggravation and slacken the muscles.

three. Gentle workout can help reduce stiffness and enhance flexibility, but it's miles essential to keep away from strenuous exercising because of the reality it is able to positioned an excessive amount of strain in your wrists. Attempt honest sports, as an instance, wrist twists, finger stretches, or hand turns, to hold your arms and wrists adaptable.

Yoga and Pilates are also extremely good low-effect wearing sports that can beautify the muscle businesses across the wrist and improve flexibility.

4. Maintain proper posture. Proper posture can assist alleviate wrist strain and prevent in addition harm. Sit at once and keep your once more directly. Adjust your pocket ebook and sit down in a chair that is supportive to keep away from awkward wrist positions.

5. Manage strain. Stress could make carpal tunnel syndrome worse by means of the use of making the ache and ache even worse. Learning pressure-relieving techniques, like contemplation, profound

breathing, or yoga, can assist with lowering feelings of anxiety and running on modern-day prosperity.

6. Change Your Sleeping Position: Sleeping in an inept feature can positioned strain on the median nerve inside the wrist, that might make Carpal Tunnel Syndrome's signs and symptoms and signs worse. To forestall this, try and lay down together along side your fingers in an independent function, making use of a wrist manual if crucial.

7. Eat nicely. A nicely-balanced weight-reduction plan can assist the frame reduce contamination and enhance favored health. Antioxidant-wealthy meals like nuts, seeds, quit result, and greens can help reduce inflammation and improve immune function.

eight. Get sufficient rest. Rest is crucial for the wrist's healing and the prevention of in addition harm.

Support businesses

Support corporations are steady locations in which dad and mom which can be going via the equal issues can percent their memories, speak about issues and approaches to cope with them, and provide every different emotional beneficial resource. Joining a help organization can assist human beings with carpal tunnel syndrome discover about new remedies, get recommendation on how to attend to themselves, and make massive connections with outstanding human beings.

Support corporations are typically supplied for gratis or at a low price and are generally led via experts inside the region. These organizations are regularly prepared with the useful resource of nonprofits, clinical facilities, or health clinics so that you can offer sufferers or the community with resources for managing their conditions. Additionally, there are numerous online help agencies that can be accessed from the advantage of one's non-public domestic, making it easy to take part even inside the face of specifically immoderate physical signs and symptoms.

Support corporations for individuals residing with carpal tunnel ailment may want to likely have precise preparations. A few gatherings might be formal, with fashionable gatherings and coordinated conversations driven via the usage of a facilitator, at the same time as others might be less prepared and 0 in more on casual sharing and mingling. Support agencies may moreover furthermore provide greater sports like workshops, exercising instructions, or even online webinars or video conferencing so that members can attend from a distance.

No do not forget what the business enterprise, guide organizations offer a blanketed, classified environment for people living with carpal tunnel syndrome to percentage their hobbies, sentiments, and encounters. When in comparison to looking to navigate their circumstance on their very non-public, individuals of manual corporations often document feeling masses tons much less remoted and further understood. Members of help corporations frequently set up close to relationships with every distinctive, enhancing a revel in of network and imparting social guide, each of that might have huge intellectual advantages.

Support agencies provide individuals with social and emotional manual in addition to sensible steerage and facts. By sharing their research with remedy and symptom manage, participants of those corporations make it much less complicated for others to get the right care. In addition to exploring self-care alternatives like physical remedy and hand-strengthening physical video games, people can advantage notion into ergonomic machine and outstanding modifications to resource the wrists and hands even as operating.

Support agencies for people residing with carpal tunnel syndrome provide many advantages and are an critical asset for people looking for profound, social, and feasible help. Joining a assist enterprise can help you find answers that provide you with the effects you want if you're struggling with this case.

Return to paintings or university

Carpal tunnel syndrome may be a crippling situation, specially for individuals who paintings or bypass to high school every day. You might experience like you may't flow returned to art work or university if you have carpal tunnel syndrome. You can, however, move again to productivity and feel confident for your potential to carry out your day-to-day obligations with the right treatments and precautions.

There are a number of treatments that could assist if carpal tunnel syndrome has been recognized. Probably the most notably identified tablets include wearing a wrist manual, taking an over the counter pain drug, and doing sports activities sports to bolster the wrist and hand muscle organizations. You may additionally moreover likewise be recommended to keep away from bodily activities that exasperate your component effects, like composing or associated with gadgets for extended time frames.